Cortisol Control
and the Beauty Connection

D0179393

Ordering

Trade bookstores in the U.S. and Canada please contact:

Publishers Group West
1700 Fourth Street, Berkeley CA 94710
Phone: (800) 788-3123   Fax: (510) 528-3444

Hunter House books are available at bulk discounts
for textbook course adoptions; to qualifying community,
health-care, and government organizations; and for special
promotions and fund-raising. For details please contact:

Special Sales Department
Hunter House Inc., PO Box 2914, Alameda CA 94501-0914
Phone: (510) 865-5282   Fax: (510) 865-4295
E-mail: ordering@hunterhouse.com

Individuals can order our books from most bookstores,
by calling (800) 266-5592, or from our website at
www.hunterhouse.com

Cortisol Control and the *Beauty* Connection

. . . .

THE ALL-NATURAL, INSIDE-OUT APPROACH TO REVERSING WRINKLES, PREVENTING ACNE AND IMPROVING SKIN TONE

SHAWN TALBOTT, PH.D., FACSM

Hunter House
PUBLISHERS

Copyright © 2007 by Shawn Talbott

All rights reserved. No part of this publication may be reproduced or transmitted in any form or by any means, electronic or mechanical, including photocopying and recording, or introduced into any information storage and retrieval system without the written permission of the copyright owner and the publisher of this book. Brief quotations may be used in reviews prepared for inclusion in a magazine, newspaper, or for broadcast. For further information please contact:

Hunter House Inc., Publishers
PO Box 2914
Alameda CA 94501-0914

Library of Congress Cataloging-in-Publication Data
Talbott, Shawn M.
Cortisol control and the beauty connection : the all-natural, inside-out approach to reversing wrinkles, preventing acne and improving skin tone / Shawn Talbott. — 1st ed.
p. cm.
Includes bibliographical references and index.
ISBN-13: 978-0-89793-479-4 (pbk.)
ISBN-10: 0-89793-479-2 (pbk.)
1. Skin—Care and hygiene. 2. Skin—Wrinkles. 3. Hydrocortisone—Physiological effect. 4. Beauty, Personal. I. Title.
RL87.T34 2007
646.7′26—dc22   2006033938

Project Credits
Cover Design: Brian Dittmar Graphic Design
Book Production: John McKercher
Developmental Editor: Naomi Rose
Copy Editor: Kelley Blewster
Proofreader: John David Marion
Indexer: Nancy D. Peterson
Acquisitions Editor: Jeanne Brondino
Editor: Alexandra Mummery
Senior Marketing Associate: Reina Santana
Customer Service Manager: Christina Sverdrup
Order Fulfillment: Washul Lakdhon
Administrator: Theresa Nelson
Computer Support: Peter Eichelberger
Publisher: Kiran S. Rana

Printed and Bound by Transcontinental Printing

Printed in Canada

9 8 7 6 5 4 3 2 1   First Edition   07 08 09 10 11

Contents

IMPORTANT NOTE

The material in this book is intended to provide a review of information regarding how caring for your skin from the inside out—especially learning to reduce stress through lifestyle changes, nutrition, supplements, and exercise—will have a beneficial effect on your skin health and skin care. Every effort has been made to provide accurate and dependable information. The contents of this book have been compiled through professional research and in consultation with medical professionals. However, health-care professionals have differing opinions, and advances in medical and scientific research are made very quickly, so some of the information may become outdated.

Therefore, the publisher, authors, and editors, as well as the professionals quoted in the book, cannot be held responsible for any error, omission, or dated material. The authors and publisher assume no responsibility for any outcome of applying the information in this book in a program of self-care or under the care of a licensed practitioner. If you have questions concerning your diet or health, or about the application of the information described in this book, consult a qualified health-care professional.

skin-care products that promise antiaging and anti-acne miracles. Turn on the TV and, while watching your favorite shows, count the number of commercials for skin-care products that claim to be able to make you look like the models who are using them. Go to any department store or skin-care boutique and note the enormous number and variety of skin-care products, each claiming a different, much-needed, and alluring result and offering a bewildering choice of what to buy, for what purpose, with what ingredients, and at what price (sometimes the higher the price, the greater the allure). Americans spend hundreds of millions of dollars every year on lotions, creams, and coatings to be applied to the surface (the dead part) of the skin. Many of these concoctions do a wonderful job of smoothing out wrinkles and giving the *appearance* of younger, healthier skin. The illusion of healthier skin, however, rapidly fades when the beauty cream wears off—not to mention that none of these products can help you *feel* better in terms of energy levels or emotional outlook. Then there are the nontopical solutions: injections such as Botox, offering a blank screen of a face to women who may feel pressured by the media, their peers, and the fear of no longer having a presence in the culture if a smile line graces their face. The most invasive solution is plastic surgery. It may produce a dramatically new look on the outside, but it costs—in money, in time required to heal, in the potential need for repeat treatments over the years, and in the unexpected gap between "I look so great on the outside, how come I don't feel different on the inside?"

The road to beautiful, healthy, glowing, youthful skin is far easier and effective than all this. Why not beautify your skin from the inside? Clearing up problem skin and reversing the aging process don't require spending a small (or large) fortune. You can depend on yourself and work with what's inside you rather than being at the mercy of external products and processes. Simply knowing about four basic aspects of how your body works and giving them what they need to function optimally—a program I call "FACE"—will free you from unwanted outside influences, put much of your money back in your pocket, and give you the most beautiful skin you've ever had. And if this weren't enough, following my FACE program will also help you lose weight, gain energy, live a more relaxed and happy life, and develop a way of eating that's as close to you, and as natural, as the palm of your hand.

What's the secret to this "magic"? It is understanding cortisol control and the beauty connection, and then taking appropriate action.

THE EFFECT OF CORTISOL CONTROL AND COLLAGEN ON A BEAUTIFUL FACE

Why is it important to control cortisol? Well, cortisol is the primary hormone that our bodies secrete when we are under stress. This means that whenever we're under stress, we're exposed to cortisol. Cortisol isn't bad in and of itself. It's a normal part of our physiological makeup. The problem occurs when we're exposed to *too much* of it on a *chronic* basis—a scenario that is all too common in today's fast-paced, overbooked way of living.

Because of cortisol's wide-ranging influence on other important aspects of metabolism (especially those metabolic pathways associated most closely with "aging"), it is often called the "death hormone." This is a fairly accurate nickname: Cortisol is a hormone that tends to increase with age, and our increased exposure to cortisol as we age has been linked to breakdown and dysfunction in every tissue in the body. This breakdown of our tissue does, in a real sense, bring us closer to death and age us unnecessarily before our time. So whether we're talking about skin or heart muscle or brain neurons, it makes sense to address cortisol as sort of a master switch in the metabolism of aging.

To learn more about how controlling cortisol can help you lose weight and combat stress and illness, my previous books on the subject, *The Cortisol Connection: Why Stress Makes You Fat and Ruins Your Health — and What You Can Do about It* (2002) and *The Cortisol Connection Diet: The Breakthrough Program to Control Stress and Lose Weight* (2004), are essential reading. They provide guidelines similar to those provided in this book, but they go into greater detail about the science behind the negative effects of cortisol on the body and the many positive effects that controlling cortisol can have on our overall well-being and in preventing illnesses such as obesity, diabetes, hypertension, osteoporosis, and syndrome X. Furthermore, *The Cortisol Connection Diet* provides a clear diet and exercise plan that will teach you how to use food and supplements to control cortisol, blood sugar, and your metabolism.

Since cortisol is basically the controller of the four metabolic pathways in the FACE program described in this book, *we* need to control *it* in order to slow down the skin's aging process, treat and prevent problem skin, and promote radiant, healthy skin. When we do this, we get unexpected perks: Controlling cortisol also produces beneficial results in terms of weight loss, improved mood, and enhanced libido! This is not to say that cortisol is the only metabolic pathway that needs to be addressed in order to promote healthy skin, but considering its profound effect on the body's functioning, cortisol control is the most logical place to start.

One major way that cortisol earns its tag as the death hormone is through its destructive effect on collagen, the most abundant protein in the human body (about a third of all the proteins) and the chief structural component of skin tissues (about 90 percent). Collagen serves as the primary framework on which all the major structures in our body, including our skin, are built. It's what wards off lines and wrinkles, and it is about the closest thing we have to a fountain of youth.

The health of our skin and bones is affected by how well we *metabolize* collagen—that is, how well our systems make collagen available to our bodies for productive use. Collagen metabolism can be influenced by our eating habits, exercise patterns, and lifestyles. When we are under stress (and this even includes the "stress" of dieting), our cortisol levels increase, contributing to a faster breakdown of tissues that contain collagen, such as bone and skin.

Another source of collagen destruction is the drying-out process that comes with aging. However, there are ways to reduce this destruction and promote the synthesis of stronger collagen fibers. Most people try to do this by using topical cosmetics that deliver lubricants and moisturizers back to the surface of the skin in an attempt to slow the aging process. Some of these topical remedies are natural and work well with the body's own self-healing tendency, as you will learn in Chapter 11, "Putting It All Together." However, the entire premise of this book is that the best, most natural way to care for your skin is to provide nourishment from the *inside*. Through stress-reduction changes in lifestyle, balanced nutrition, dietary supplements, and exercise, you can control the amount of cortisol that gets released into your bloodstream during stress. Doing this can greatly help bring the collagen-turnover process into balance, and it can even tip the scales slightly in your favor when it comes to repairing vital connective tissues and preventing (or at least delaying) some of the conditions that we normally associate with aging.

If you are still too young to require antiaging advice and your concern is treating and preventing problem skin—for example, if your situation is not dry skin but the opposite: oily, acne-prone skin—my FACE program will start you on a regimen of inside-out skin care while you are young. Since this is a program that makes you *feel* better as well as *look* better, it can grow with you very comfortably through the years, so that when your skin becomes more mature, it will have the long-term benefit of the FACE foundation.

THE "FACE" PROGRAM

FACE is an acronym for Free radicals, Advanced glycation end-products (AGEs), Cortisol, and Eicosanoids. (Free radicals have to do with oxidation, AGEs with blood-sugar levels, and eicosanoids with inflammation.) Each of these complicated-sounding topics is explained in the book.

The premise of the FACE program is that the outward appearance of beautiful skin starts on the inside, and that wrinkled, blemished skin is *not* an inevitable result of aging. Nor is problem skin something that can only be dealt with by expensive, often abrasive outside-in means. This all-natural approach to beautiful skin and a youthful complexion is based on the latest scientific evidence and years of real-life experience with hundreds of participants. As you learn about and follow the guidance of the FACE program, *your* face will become more and more naturally beautiful.

What we perceive as aging is actually a complicated and multifaceted phenomenon related to skin breakdown and repair—a cyclical process that we scientists refer to as "tissue turnover." In the case of skin, we call it "collagen turnover." The most effective solution to a multifaceted *problem* is a multifaceted *program*, and that's exactly what the FACE program is. Not only is it simple and inexpensive to follow, but you'll find that it's nothing short of miraculous in the way it makes you look, feel, and function.

The reason why controlling cortisol is so important for healthy skin is because stress and cortisol exposure can set off higher FACE levels. This sets in motion bodily processes that run counter to healthy skin, such as

- increased appetite for sweets, leading to glycation, collagen breakdown, and wrinkles

- increased oil production in the skin, leading to acne
- increased production of eicosanoids and related cyto-kines, leading to reduced wound healing, slower skin re-generation, and more redness, itchiness, and swelling
- free-radical load, leading to skin microdamage and loss of skin moisture and skin-barrier protection, and inter-fering with insulin function, thus increasing blood-sugar levels and glycation

Fortunately, the FACE program offers a skin- and colla-gen-specific approach that builds whole-body, systemic bene-fits. This means that in addition to the benefits of a targeted skin-health regimen (including reduced wrinkles and blem-ishes), you will also experience reduced stress, better mood, less body fat, improved muscle tone, and many other unex-pected and welcome results.

MAKING SENSE OF THE "FACE" PROGRAM
HOW I CAME TO DISCOVER
THE IMPORTANCE OF CORTISOL CONTROL

I never set out to write a book about beauty—or about skin health for that matter. Many years ago, when I was a young Ph.D. student at Rutgers University, my focus was on bone metabolism—specifically, on uncovering the complex inter-actions between nutrition, lifestyle, and osteoporosis. In our lab, we studied the interplay of diet and exercise on collagen. Through our studies and those of our scientific colleagues, we came to understand that collagen metabolism (and thus the health of our skin and bones) can be influenced by the world around us. Our lab was among the first in the world to show that the "stress" of dieting for weight loss increased cortisol levels and contributed to a faster breakdown of collagen-con-taining tissues, such as bone and skin.

Today, the scientific community accepts the fact that chronic stress and overexposure to cortisol leads to rapid breakdown in other tissues, including brain neurons, blood vessels, muscles, immune cells, and many more. Because collagen is the chief protein in skin, this cortisol-induced acceleration of collagen breakdown inevitably leads to skin problems, including wrinkles, acne, and uneven skin tone. Collagen breakdown and skin damage can also be hastened by other factors, including metabolic processes, such as inflammation, oxidation, and glycation. Imbalances in each of these four processes are well documented in the scientific and medical literature as resulting in the rapid and dramatic effects that we view as premature aging.

However, until I conducted a particular weight-loss program, none of this had any direct meaning for me. I am not a dermatologist but a nutritional biochemist, trained in sports medicine, health management, and exercise physiology. For the last decade or so, my career has been focused on using nutrition and other lifestyle strategies to help people lose weight and improve their health. To this end, I designed and conducted a series of popular and very successful weight-loss programs. They generally run three or four times each year, and we always have a waiting list. They take place near Salt Lake City, Utah, where I now live with my wife and two children.

These programs follow a regimen that I call the SENSE program, because it incorporates Stress management, Exercise, Nutrition, Supplementation, and Evaluation. Participants invariably experience fat loss, muscle gain, increased energy, improved mood, reduced stress, elevated libido, and a host of related benefits. Best of all, our participants never feel deprived, hungry, or as though they are following a "diet." In fact, in the early weeks of each session, there are always several participants who declare that the program will never work for them because it's "too easy." Our response is always the same:

"Trust us," we say. "Just stick with the program for a few weeks, and you'll see the benefits." They do—and they're amazed.

My discovery of the cortisol/beauty connection was something of an accident. During the first few years that we were running the SENSE weight-loss programs, participants would comment that they "felt great" and thought they "looked better." At first, my staff and I always interpreted those positive comments as a reflection of these participants' excitement about finally being able to lose weight and keep it off. Eventually, however, it dawned on us that there might be something more at work here.

We got this "sense" when we recruited a group of participants, who were already fit and lean, to see whether our SENSE program could help them control their perception of stress relative to eating during a traditionally high-stress period of time (the holiday season from Thanksgiving to New Year's Day). These mostly young, good-looking, successful men and women didn't have very much weight to lose; they simply got stressed out during the holidays and gained weight as a result of stress eating.

After they finished the program, they *also* told us that they felt and looked better, which we found very interesting. We could understand the "feel better" part, because we discovered that their stress and cortisol levels were reduced by about 20 percent after they'd followed the SENSE program. But the "look better" part was a surprise (remember, these folks already looked pretty darn good). Our unexpected discovery was that the same SENSE program that made them feel less stressed out (and that had helped previous overweight participants lose weight) was also delivering some very noticeable beauty benefits. Our participants found that by controlling their stress levels they were also controlling their exposure to cortisol. As a result, their wrinkles were reduced, their skin wasn't breaking out, and their skin (especially facial skin) was clearer, smoother, and more youthful in appearance. Another interesting finding that went hand-in-hand with looking and feeling better was that their sex drive (libido) was improved. (Needless to say, this freaked out the parents in the program whose teenagers were participating and grossed out the teens in the program whose parents were participating.)

It turns out that all these effects—from weight loss to enhanced mood to healthy skin to improved libido—are the result of controlling cortisol. However, when we explained the cortisol connection in proper, scientifically sound, and rational terms, our participants insisted on referring to the program as the "fountain-of-youth class."

FACING YOUR BEAUTIFUL FUTURE

The FACE program that you will read about in this book is an updated version of the popular SENSE weight-loss program, and it is the *only* comprehensive program that controls all four of the F-A-C-E aspects that cause accelerated, premature aging. FACE builds on the whole-body, systemic benefits of SENSE, using a skin- and collagen-specific approach to meet your unique skin-care needs. This means that in following the FACE program, you will realize every one of the benefits that our participants in the SENSE program enjoyed—reduced stress, better mood, less body fat, improved muscle tone, and more—but with the added benefit of having a targeted skin-health regimen that will reduce wrinkles, blemishes, and problem skin.

Let me tell you what to expect with *Cortisol Control and the Beauty Connection.* Part I gives you the science behind the FACE program so you can understand what goes on under your skin.

- *Chapter 1* provides an overview of the FACE Program— my comprehensive metabolic approach to unifying the four primary, scientifically based antiaging theories into a single, easy-to-follow, realistic program.

- *Chapter* 2 provides a science-based overview of collagen and normal skin metabolism—how it should work, what it should look like, and what is going on under the surface of your body's largest organ.

- *Chapter* 3 delves into the "aging" process and its reversal through the FACE program, and it demystifies the metabolic process that our skin undergoes every hour of every day. By understanding a bit of the metabolism behind "normal" skin and "aging" skin, you can gain a deeper understanding of the hows and whys of FACE and how it can work for you.

- *Chapter* 4 discusses some of the primary causes and solutions behind our most prevalent skin issues: wrinkles, acne and blemishes, and uneven skin tone, including redness, rosacea, and blotches.

Part II gives you specific dietary information that you can follow to feed your FACE.

- *Chapter* 5 presents the Helping Hand diet, so named because you use the size of your hand as a portion-control device. This lets you balance your intake of carbohydrate, protein, fat, and fiber in a way that considers both the quantity and quality of the foods you eat.

- *Chapter* 6 discusses supplements you can take to *control cortisol* (the "C" of FACE), including ashwagandha, cordyceps, epimedium, damiana, magnolia bark, kava kava, ginseng, passionflower, *Rhodiola rosea*, schisandra, valerian, and theanine.

- *Chapter* 7 discusses supplements you can take to *control oxidation* (the "F"—for "free radicals"—of FACE).

These include vitamin A, spirulina, vitamin C, vitamin E, beta-carotene, green tea, flavonoids/polyphenols, lycopene, lutein/zeaxanthin, and gotu kola.

- *Chapter 8* discusses supplements you can take to *control AGEs* (the "A" of FACE)—that is, to control blood sugar. These include chromium, vanadium, zinc, alpha-lipoic acid, *Gymnema sylvestre*, banaba leaf, bitter melon, panax ginseng, and fenugreek.

- *Chapter 9* discusses supplements you can take to *control eicosanoids* (the "E" of FACE)—that is, the effects of inflammation. These include essential fatty acids, evening primrose oil, borage oil, *Boswellia serrata*, bromelain and papain, flaxseed oil, ginger, and white willow bark.

- *Chapter 10* gives you a step-by-step guide to starting and following the FACE program.

- *Chapter 11* puts it all together with advice from various skin-care experts on how to care naturally for your most extensive, sensitive, exquisite organ—your skin.

- Finally, you will find appendixes containing recipes and exercises, and a Resources section listing contact information for the various sources mentioned in the book.

I hope that you're looking forward to starting your own FACE program. As an active researcher, and as someone who likes to apply science to help people and to "practice what I preach," I invite you to share your thoughts about *Cortisol Control and the Beauty Connection* and your experiences with the FACE program. Please feel free to e-mail me at www.cortisolconnection.com. I look forward to hearing from you.

PART I

The

Science Behind

Inside-Out Skin Care

and the

FACE Program

. . . .
. . .
. .
. .

CHAPTER 1

An Overview
of the
FACE Program

The longer I live, the more beautiful life becomes.
If you foolishly ignore beauty, you will soon find yourself
without it. Your life will be impoverished. But if you invest in
beauty, it will remain with you all the days of your life.

— Frank Lloyd Wright
American architect, 1867–1959

If you're wondering what the FACE program is all about, I can sum it up for you in a single sentence: The outward appearance of beautiful skin *starts on the inside*, and wrinkled, blemished skin does *not* have to be an inevitable result of aging. FACE, as you discovered in the Introduction, is an acronym for Free radicals, Advanced glycation end-products (AGEs), Cortisol, and Eicosanoids—bodily processes that need to be understood and controlled in order to protect the health of your skin and total body. Fortunately, this is what the FACE program does so successfully. As a multipronged approach to simultaneously addressing multiple causes of aging, this program can in many ways be thought of as a "Unified Theory of Aging."

GOOD REASONS TO SIGN UP
FOR THE FACE PROGRAM

Considering all the "miraculous" antiaging solutions that are vying for your attention, what's the advantage of giving the FACE program a try? Because it's the only truly *comprehensive* approach to ultimate skin health. Also, the FACE program does not claim that there is one single "aging demon," the control of which will do everything for everyone.

For example, some popular antiwrinkle programs focus on controlling inflammation. Although this is a great place to start, inflammation is only *one* of the primary causes of premature aging; therefore, inflammation-control programs are automatically limited in their overall effects and benefits. Then there are the anti-acne programs that focus only on slathering the skin with topical creams to control pimples—but do nothing to modulate the day-to-day skin metabolism that leads to acne in the first place. Likewise there are antiaging programs that focus on controlling free radicals with topical antioxidant creams or supplements, or that focus only on controlling glycation by eating less sugar and by eating foods with a lower glycemic index. The result? Limited programs with limited focus lead to limited benefits for *you*.

I'm not against all such programs. I think many of them offer some hope and some help. But why give yourself less than the whole solution? Why would you choose a program that was more complicated to follow and more limited in scope, when the FACE program enables you to control *all four* metabolic aspects of aging *at the same time* with a single, easy-to-follow regimen?

GETTING TO THE ROOTS
OF THE SKIN-DAMAGE CYCLE

Being more than skin deep, the FACE program nourishes your skin by getting to the *roots* of the skin-damage cycle.

Scientists and doctors both agree that excessive **inflammation** (which is caused by eicosanoids and cytokines) can lead to accelerated skin damage and breakdown, so it makes a lot of sense to control inflammation to promote skin health. But if we look deeper to find the *causes* of inflammation, we quickly see other factors that we can control. Since **oxidation** (which is caused by free radicals) leads to inflammation at the cellular level, why not control oxidation? Great idea—but why not look even further up the metabolic chain of events to see if we can control or modulate the causes of oxidation.

When we do this, we see that **glycation** (cellular damage caused by sugars) can lead to oxidation (which can, in turn, lead to inflammation)—so we have another factor that we can address. Should we stop there? Of course not, because when we look even higher up the metabolic stream, we see that **stress** (and the cortisol exposure that stress causes) can lead to glycation, which can lead to oxidation, which in turn leads to inflammation. Unfortunately, we don't currently know enough from scientific or medical research to go any further "upstream" with regard to the metabolic control of cellular aging. Stress is as far upstream as we can go at this time—but that's still pretty good.

This gives us four aspects of metabolism that we can address to control skin structure and function—and, therefore, appearance. Perhaps the best news of all is that each of these four aspects of metabolism is easily controlled by factors related to lifestyle: diet, exercise, stress management, and the use of natural products, such as supplements and topicals.

WHAT IS "FACE"?

As I've mentioned, the acronym "FACE" stands for the four principal metabolic aspects of aging:

F = Free Radicals
This is where oxidation comes in. Free radicals are highly reactive forms of oxygen that can damage cell membranes and

other cellular structures throughout the body—but especially in the skin. Free radicals come at us from internal sources, such as breathing and metabolizing food into energy, as well as from external sources, such as sunlight and air pollution. Luckily, we can control free-radical exposure and the cellular damage (termed "oxidation") that it causes through the antioxidant recommendations in the FACE program, which are discussed in Chapter 7.

A = Advanced Glycation End-Products (AGEs)

The abbreviation "AGEs" says it all. Advanced glycation makes you look older. Glycation is the process by which sugar molecules become attached to protein molecules and inhibit their normal functioning. Too much sugar—or, more precisely, poor control of blood sugar—can lead rapidly to an accumulation of glycated proteins, with the end result being skin problems such as increased wrinkles, swelling, redness, and acne. As with the control of free radicals described above, the nutritional recommendations in the FACE program are designed to control blood sugar by modulating the function and activity of insulin (the hormone responsible for regulating blood sugar). These recommendations are presented in Chapter 8.

C = Cortisol

Cortisol, as explained in the Introduction, is the body's primary stress hormone. So whenever we're under stress, we're exposed to cortisol. Cortisol production in the body is a normal part of human life. It only becomes a problem when we're exposed to too much of it on a chronic basis—a scenario that is simply all too common in the hurry-hurry, always "on" world of the twenty-first century. Cortisol overexposure leads invariably to increases in inflammation (see below), oxidation, and glycation. In many ways, cortisol is the "master controller" among the four metabolic pathways addressed by the FACE program, so while the biggest bang for your buck in terms of promoting skin health will come from controlling cortisol (and by default, controlling the other aspects of skin aging), it makes sense to simultaneously control the other aspects in order to create a truly comprehensive approach. Recommendations for controlling cortisol are presented in Chapter 6.

E = Eicosanoids

The function of these inflammatory molecules (sometimes referred to as cytokines) is to regulate inflammation. Inflammation is a normal metabolic process with some life-sustaining benefits. For example, without a robust inflammatory process, we'd quickly succumb to bacterial and viral infections. However, when the inflammatory response becomes overactive (as it can with allergies and with some forms of heart disease) or misdirected (such as when it leads to more skin damage instead of less), we need to rebalance the inflammatory cascade back toward its natural anti-inflammatory mode. The FACE program not only helps to control inflammation directly (by modulating eicosanoids), it also helps to balance free radicals, AGEs, and cortisol—three aspects of metabolism that can lead to hyperinflammation when left unchecked. Recommendations for controlling eicosanoids are presented in Chapter 9.

"FACE" IN ACTION

You've heard the saying "You are what you eat." But did you ever stop to think that what you eat might also influence how you *look*? Based on several recent scientific studies and many decades of population studies, we now know quite clearly that nutritional factors can influence skin health in a variety of ways. For example, your choice of diet can promote or prevent many of the metabolic factors associated with acne, wrinkles, discoloration, and the very process of skin aging itself. The following is a summary of dietary actions called for in the FACE program. Each of these topics is discussed in more detail in later chapters.

What Not to Eat

When it comes to diet and skin health, we know a great deal about what *not* to do. This boils down to avoiding or limiting your intake of highly refined carbohydrates, sodas, and processed foods containing high-fructose corn syrup and transfats (the label will say "hydrogenated oil" or "partially hydrogenated oil"). Why do you need to avoid these types of highly processed foods? Because they set off a metabolic chain reaction in the body that leads to unhealthy elevations in blood sugar, insulin, cortisol, cytokines, and free radicals. Yikes!

Not only are these metabolic events bad for your long-term health, they're also bad for both your long- and short-term *appearance*. For example, chowing down on that monster-sized, white-flour bagel (which contains lots of refined carbs) leads to microscopic tissue destruction via a number of related events, including:

- Spikes in blood-sugar and insulin levels, which lead to protein glycation and destruction of collagen and elastin (key structural proteins in healthy skin)
- Elevated cortisol levels, which lead to imbalances in the inflammatory process in favor of proinflammatory eicosanoids (which lead to swelling, redness, and further tissue damage)
- Inflammatory eicosanoid signaling, which elevates free-radical destruction of tissue membranes throughout the body—especially in the skin

What's Good to Eat

It's not a pleasant thought that poor dietary choices can lead to so much destructive metabolism in your body. But all of us make these choices many times a day—indeed, every time we eat! Luckily, the availability of very good scientific evidence can help us choose a diet providing ingredients that will not only reduce these detrimental metabolic chain reactions but actually prevent and reverse the effects on skin health caused by glycation, inflammation, and all the rest.

Here are some of the easiest ways to control these metabolic marauders:

- Eat more of the right kinds of fats (and less of the bad kind).
- Eat fewer refined carbohydrates (and more whole-grain carbs).
- Eat more antioxidants (found in brightly colored fruits/veggies) and use supplements.
- Reduce stress (or control your exposure to the stress hormone cortisol).

Good Fats, Good Carbs

The type of fat and the type of carbohydrate that you eat are vitally important in determining your overall level of inflammation and ultimate risk for heart disease. This information is based on very convincing data collected on more than ninety thousand women and fifty thousand men by researchers at Harvard University since the mid-1970s. Their recommendations in dietary choices focus on healthy fats (olive, canola, soy, corn, sunflower, and peanut oils) and healthy carbohydrates (whole-grain foods such as whole-wheat bread, oatmeal, and brown rice), and the consumption of these is associated with a 30–40 percent reduction in risk for inflammatory heart disease. And eating more monounsaturated oils is associated with better hydration and pH of the skin, according to a recent study by Dutch researchers, published in the *American Journal of Clinical Nutrition* (February 2003), which supports the Harvard recommendations. Additionally, the astonishing differences in acne rates between populations eating a high intake of refined carbohydrates (adult acne rates as high as 40–54 percent) and populations eating fewer refined carbs (virtually zero adult acne) have been noted by researchers from the University of Colorado in the *Archives of Dermatology* (2002).

Modern diets supply roughly twenty to twenty-five times more omega-6 fatty acids than omega-3 fatty acids. This situation predisposes our bodies toward proinflammatory cytokines and systemic inflammation. The best way to address this imbalance is to limit your intake of omega-6 fats (especially fried foods; for more information see Chapter 9) while simultaneously increasing your consumption of omega-3 fats—for example, by eating fatty fish such as salmon, mackerel, and bluefish. For people who can't or don't want to eat more fatty fish, a daily fish oil supplement can provide the omega-3s needed to help quell inflammatory cytokines. A number of studies have shown that the anti-inflammatory properties of dietary omega-3 fatty acids can help to modulate skin inflammation.

Brighter Is Better

Be sure to include representatives of the entire antioxidant network (vitamins C and E, thiols, carotenoids, and flavonoids). Korean researchers have reported in the *Annals of the New York Academy of Sciences* (2001) that free radicals are intimately involved in the inflammatory process that leads to accelerated skin aging. Choose brightly colored fruits and vegetables, such as berries, tomatoes, and carrots, for the highest content of carotenoids and flavonoids. When supplementing, avoid megadoses of single antioxidant compounds and focus instead on selecting products that provide a balanced blend from among each category of the antioxidant network.

Stress Less

Cortisol is elevated in response to stressful events, a lack of sleep, and even dieting. Researchers in London have reported in the *Journal of the American Heart Association* that even short periods of stress can increase levels of cortisol and cyto-kines in the blood—and those elevated cortisol/cytokine levels have been associated with development of the inflammatory "metabolic syndrome," a cluster of symptoms including obe-sity, diabetes, hypertension, and elevated cholesterol (*Circula-tion* 2002). Effective cortisol control can be achieved by bal-ancing carbohydrate intake with proteins and healthy fats and by adding a variety of dietary supplements to your daily regi-men—for example, theanine, beta-sitosterol, and adaptogens such as cordyceps, ginseng, rhodiola, and others. In later chap-ters of this book, you'll find many valuable stress-reducing rec-ommendations within the FACE program. In Chapter 11 in particular, our panel of skin-care experts touches on the im-portance of mindset and attitude in controlling stress.

A CONCLUDING WORD

As you can see, just as we *are* what we eat, in very general terms we also tend to *look like* what we eat! And who wants to look like junk? The solution is to FACE the nutritional facts and eat your way to healthy skin by focusing on healthy carbs and fats, controlling stress and cortisol, and including enough antioxi-dants and omega-3 fatty acids in your daily diet. In this way, you can truly achieve health and beauty from the inside out.

As discussed above, there is nothing wrong with following an antiwrinkle program based on "just" inflammatory control or "just" free-radical control. You'll undoubtedly see benefits from the age-old "salad and salmon" diets advocated by many dermatologists. However, as with all complicated scenarios, if your solution to a complex problem is too simple, then you're bound to spin your wheels and your results are likely to be limited. Such is the case with existing (limited) programs: You may be controlling inflammation, but you're losing ground to oxidation; and, while you're controlling oxidation, you're losing ground to glycation, and so on. The FACE program treats skin health from the perspective of *metabolic control,* and by addressing the cellular and hormonal aspects of skin metabolism, it gets right to the root of the problem.

. . . .
.
.

CHAPTER 2

What's Happening under the Skin: The Collagen Story

Nature gives you the face you have at twenty;
it is up to you to merit the face you have at fifty.

— Coco Chanel
French fashion designer, 1883–1971

Quick—name the largest organ in the body. Liver? Nope. Intestines? Close, but no. Brain? Forget about it. The correct answer is the skin. It may be hard to imagine, but the skin isn't just a layer of dead cells. Underneath that first layer of epidermis (which *is* composed of dead skin cells) lie several thicker layers of living dermis and subcutaneous tissues.

Okay, so skin is your body's largest organ. It's your first line of defense against the outside world, and it encompasses a vast network of blood vessels, nerves, and glands (for sweat and oil). The average person's skin covers about twenty-five square feet and weighs more than six pounds when properly hydrated (more on this later).

Your skin offers you more protection than you may think. Aside from affording protection for underlying tissues and organs, harmful light rays, and disease-causing infectious agents, your skin also assists in controlling body temperature, prevents excessive loss of vitamins and minerals, receives sensory input from the environment, excretes water and salts, and synthesizes many important compounds, including vitamin D. What a busy, helpful organ!

THE STRUCTURE OF THE SKIN

Structurally, skin is composed of two primary parts: the outer, thinner portion called the *epidermis* and the deeper, thicker connective-tissue layer called the *dermis*. Beneath these two layers of skin lie *subcutaneous tissues*, including adipose tissue, or fat. Fibers from the dermis extend downward to anchor the skin to the subcutaneous layers. In turn, the subcutaneous layers are firmly attached to even deeper tissues and organs.

Although the skin is about 60 percent water, the remaining "dry" portion is mostly composed of three types of protein that play critical roles in skin structure and health. A great deal of what causes the skin to wrinkle stems from problems with building and maintaining this network of three skin proteins:

1. **Keratin,** your skin's strongest protein, is found in the outer epidermis layer and is responsible for skin rigidity.

2. **Collagen,** which is found in the dermis, is the most abundant protein, comprising roughly 90 percent of skin tissue. Collagen is about the closest thing we have to a fountain of youth since it wards off lines and wrinkles.

3. **Elastin,** collagen's protein buddy and also found in the dermis, is the elastic that gives skin its structure. It is diminished levels of elastin that can cause your skin to sag.

HAIR AND NAILS
WHERE COLLAGEN GOES TO DIE

Why doesn't it hurt to get a haircut or to clip your fingernails? Many people might automatically answer that hair and nails have no feeling because they are "dead." A more accurate answer would be that hair and nails have no nerve endings, and thus they don't receive or perceive painful stimuli. To think about this question in another way, ask, "Why does it hurt if you have your hair pulled?" The answer is because the hair is being detached from its "living" attachment in the skin.

The cells that make up hair and nail tissue originate in and receive support from the healthy collagen fibers in the skin matrix. As the hair and nail cells accumulate, the interior of each cell is slowly replaced with keratin, a protein very similar to collagen. We know from decades of research in humans and animals that supporting collagen metabolism with diet and exercise can help support the process of hair and nail growth "from the inside"—by supporting the early steps of collagen and keratin formation.

What we know as "aging" is really the outward observation of an imbalance between collagen breakdown and repair—and the interplay of oxidation, inflammation, glycation, and stress that governs that process.

COLLAGEN TURNOVER
A NATURAL PROCESS WORTH SUPPORTING

Collagen is continually undergoing a process of breakdown and repair. This cycle, referred to as "turnover," is a perfectly normal part of keeping the collagen at its peak health. The turnover process allows tissues with a high collagen content—such as skin—to adapt to stress and to repair themselves after suffering damage. For instance, let's say you overdo it at the company softball game and wake up the next morning with stiff, achy muscles and joints. The pain and discomfort you feel result from damage to your muscles, tendons, and ligaments (all rich in collagen, just like your skin) caused by the stress of overexertion. You already know that the pain and stiffness will fade away over the next couple of days. Why this will take place is because your natural turnover process will begin to remove the damaged tissue and replace it with brand-new healthy tissue that is just a little bit stronger than it was before.

The collagen turnover process in skin and other tissues can be influenced by a variety of factors, including age, physical health, and nutrient intake. It doesn't take a rocket scientist to point out the wrinkling of skin, the stiffening of joints, and the graying (or loss) of hair as we age. We've known for decades that regular physical activity and proper nutrition can help delay or reverse some of the deterioration of our bodies. In fact, many of the losses in function considered to be "inevitable" consequences of aging are little more than minor inefficiencies and subtle deficits in this turnover process that have built up over many years.

For example, joint stiffness is probably the first noticeable consequence of aging. You may try to get up from the chair or carry something across the yard and find yourself admitting, "Whoa, I never felt *that* before." What you're feeling in this situation is the result of years and years of accumulated stress (and inadequate repair) in your connective tissue. Well, the very same process is at work in your skin—and the key to maintaining optimal tissue function is to maintain and support the naturally balanced process of collagen turnover.

Virtually every situation that we associate with "aging" can be directly attributed to the lifetime balance of degradation and repair within each tissue. In the innumerable cases that make us feel older (for example, joint pain, weak muscles, stiff tendons and ligaments), there is a significant underlying connection to collagen health. In each case, the balance between breakdown and repair has tilted in favor of collagen loss.

Even if collagen breakdown outpaces repair by just a very slight amount, the combined effect over the years will lead to dysfunction. If you could just give the balance a little bump—and either nudge the synthesis of collagen a little higher or push the breakdown of collagen a little lower—then you'd be back in balance. Even better, if you could stack the deck in your favor by increasing collagen synthesis above the breakdown rate, then you could actually make *gains* in those areas that previously gave you grief.

That's what the FACE program can help you do: tilt the balance of collagen breakdown and repair back into your favor by controlling oxidation, inflammation, glycation, and stress (the key regulators of collagen metabolism).

COLLAGEN: THE STRUCTURE FOR LIFE

As mentioned previously, collagen is a protein. All proteins are a collection of smaller building blocks called *amino acids*. These amino acids are held together by various chemical inter-actions, which cause the formation of small groups called *peptides* and then larger groups called *proteins* (see Figure 2.1). Every protein in the body has a specific and essential function; there are no "extra" proteins. For example, some proteins per-form specialized functions, such as digestion, in which pro-teins called *enzymes* break food down into smaller and smaller

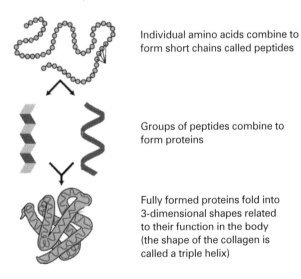

Individual amino acids combine to form short chains called peptides

Groups of peptides combine to form proteins

Fully formed proteins fold into 3-dimensional shapes related to their function in the body (the shape of the collagen is called a triple helix)

Figure 2.1: Amino acid and protein structure

pieces for absorption by the stomach and the intestines. Other enzymatic proteins are involved in metabolism, as they help to convert food into energy. These types of proteins are sometimes referred to as "functional" proteins because they perform highly specialized functions.

Functional proteins are often so specialized that they can only do one very specific task (although they typically do it very well). For example, the protein that helps us store fat in our cells can *only* do storage. A completely different protein is needed to help the cells *release* that same fat, and yet another protein is needed to help *break down* that fat for energy. It sounds complicated to have thousands of different proteins to perform thousands of different functions (and it is!), but it makes a lot of sense. After all, you wouldn't want some general-function enzyme running around your body turning a process on over here and another process off over there. Your metabolism would be in complete chaos!

Other proteins play a *structural* role in the body; that is, they provide a framework or foundation on which our bodies are built. Collagen is the most abundant protein in the human body, accounting for about a third of all the proteins. Collagen serves as the primary framework—or basement layer—on which all the major structures in our bodies are built. In many ways, collagen can be thought of as the "steel girders" on which the rest of your body (including your skin) is built.

As with other proteins, the collagen molecule is a long string of individual amino acid building blocks. The collagen molecules take the form of very long strands—much longer than most other proteins. These strands are wound around each other like a rope, in groups of three, to form a structure called a triple helix (see Figure 2.2 on the next page). The triple helix arrangement gives collagen many of its properties, such as strength, flexibility, and toughness, and it allows collagen to be used in a wide variety of structures, including bones, joints, skin, muscles, tendons, and ligaments.

COLLAGEN MAINTENANCE
SYNTHESIS, BREAKDOWN, AND REPAIR

The process of collagen synthesis and repair involves a complex chain of events. Collagen synthesis begins deep within individual cells in each tissue. Amino acids are transported into the cell and added to the growing collagen chain—sort of like adding beads to a necklace. As the beads (amino acids) are added, the necklace (collagen molecule) gets longer. When three collagen molecules are finished, they are twisted together by a specialized group of enzymes to form a braided structure—the triple helix mentioned above. This triple helix is then transported out of the cell for further processing. Once outside the cell, various reactions—some requiring enzymes and some occurring on their own over time—help bring these triple helix collagen molecules into the proper arrangement. The entire process goes something like this:

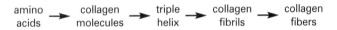

amino acids → collagen molecules → triple helix → collagen fibrils → collagen fibers

Depending on the tissue involved, the collagen molecules may be arranged in fibers placed very close together (as in bone) or spaced a little further apart (as in joint cartilage). The precise arrangement of each collagen fiber will help determine its ultimate function.

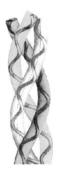

The collagen protein is comprised of three individual protein strands that are twisted together into a single structure—the triple helix—that gives collagen its unique strength and flexibility.

Figure 2.2: Collagen triple helix structure

Once the collagen fibers are in place, then the real work begins: *maintaining* this complex collagen fiber arrangement against the repetitive strain of everyday events. To help maintain its strength and resiliency, as mentioned earlier, collagen continually undergoes a process of breakdown and rebuilding. This chain of events is a recycling process that helps get rid of older collagen fibers that may be damaged or weakened and replaces them with newer, healthier collagen fibers that are stronger and more able to withstand strain. Just as public works crews are constantly being sent out to repair potholes in roads, your body has to fight an ongoing struggle to maintain and repair its collagen network.

Without this ongoing renewal and repair process of collagen turnover, small bits of daily damage would build up and result in a serious deterioration of the tissue. In joints, this might lead to painful arthritis; in bones, it might lead to a stress fracture; and in muscles and tendons, the risk for strains and tears might be increased. These are the more serious potential risks. However, there are a number of other adverse effects from an inadequate or inefficient collagen turnover process, such as premature wrinkling of skin, graying (or loss) of hair, and even premature tooth loss.

COLLAGEN AND SKIN

I certainly don't need to tell anybody reading this book that skin wrinkles as we age. Wrinkled skin is pretty much something that we've all come to accept as an inevitable part of the aging process. Have you ever stopped to wonder, though, just *why* it is that our skin wrinkles as we age? How about the fact that some people have more wrinkles than others? Can something be done about it? Happily, the answer is yes. There are a number of approaches that can be taken to help combat the appearance of wrinkles in the skin.

The basic underlying reason that our skin wrinkles with age is because we "dry out." As we age, our bodies actually lose moisture little by little, and the end result is that we "shrivel up" a bit. This drying-out process can be accelerated by environmental factors, such as prolonged exposure to the sun and smoking. Luckily, however, it can also be slowed somewhat by the wide range of topical cosmetics that deliver lubricants and moisturizers back to the surface of the skin.

A different approach to preventing the drying and wrinkling effects of aging is to moisturize the skin by providing nourishment from the inside—with balanced nutrition and dietary supplements. As we age, the deeper layer of skin, the dermis, gets thinner (see Figure 2.3). The progressive breakdown of collagen and elastin (which can be accelerated by oxidation, inflammation, glycation, and stress) results in a loss of skin strength and a reduced ability to maintain adequate levels of lubricating fluid. Proper dietary support can help to reduce the destruction of collagen and promote the synthesis of stronger collagen fibers.

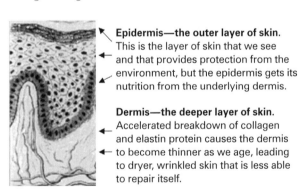

Epidermis—the outer layer of skin. This is the layer of skin that we see and that provides protection from the environment, but the epidermis gets its nutrition from the underlying dermis.

Dermis—the deeper layer of skin. Accelerated breakdown of collagen and elastin protein causes the dermis to become thinner as we age, leading to dryer, wrinkled skin that is less able to repair itself.

Figure 2.3: The structure of the skin

With age, a number of noticeable changes in collagen structures become apparent. Collagen fibers lose their elasticity, so we may become "droopy" in areas of our body that used to be firm. Collagen in skin begins to lose its ability to hold water, so our skin dries out and begins to wrinkle. The keratinized cells destined to become strands of hair become fewer in number and lose their ability to produce pigment—so hair either turns gray or it turns loose (i.e., falls out). With age, cartilage cells lose their ability to produce new collagen, so we lose cartilage thickness and our joints begin to ache. Bones become weaker over time as the rate of collagen and mineral breakdown exceeds our ability to replace losses with healthy tissue.

As a result of all these small changes in collagen-containing structures, we slowly begin to lose flexibility and mobility. The end result—which often goes unnoticed until it's too late—is that we can't get around as well as we could when we were younger (when our ability to maintain our collagen structures was better).

Again, if we could just balance the collagen turnover process—or, better yet, tip the scales slightly in our favor—we could balance out the destruction and repair of our vital connective tissues and prevent (or delay) some of the conditions that we normally associate with aging.

A CONCLUDING WORD

Now you know something about what collagen is and the important role it plays in maintaining the structural integrity of the body. You have also been introduced to the general concept of harnessing the body's own metabolic machinery to support the process of collagen repair and renewal.

To refresh your memory about some key points:

- Collagen is the chief structural protein in the body.

- Structural proteins are needed to provide organization and strength to connective tissues, such as cartilage, bones, teeth, muscles, tendons, ligaments, skin, hair, and nails.

- Collagen undergoes a continual process of synthesis, breakdown, and repair, known as "turnover."

- Collagen turnover is the body's way of removing older, weaker, damaged tissue and replacing it with newer, stronger, healthier tissue.

- The imbalance between collagen breakdown and synthesis (turnover) is the primary cause of wrinkles and problems with skin/wound healing.

- Collagen turnover can be managed by controlling oxidation, inflammation, glycation, and stress—as shown in the FACE program.

stand as "aging," each corresponding to a letter of the FACE acronym. Each of these metabolic processes can lead to accelerated aging when *unbalanced* (in a negative direction), but can also lead to a dramatic "antiaging" effect when *balanced* or only *temporarily unbalanced* (in a positive direction). In addition, each of these four aspects of metabolism is intimately intertwined and interdependent on the others. This situation can be good if you can control all four simultaneously, but it can also be very frustrating if you control one area while another area continues to cause problems.

For example, scientists have known for decades that highly reactive oxygen molecules called free radicals are a primary source of aging because they cause damage (oxidation) to cellular structures such as membranes, mitochondria, and DNA, leading to cellular dysfunction. The most viable antiaging approach would seem to be controlling free-radical metabolism. And it is—up to a point. Unfortunately, another metabolic process, inflammation (caused by eicosanoids), can also accelerate cellular damage and aging. Even worse, oxidation can lead to inflammation, and vice versa. Adding to the confusion is the recent scientific understanding that inflammatory control is tightly linked to glucose levels in the blood—meaning that fluctuations in blood sugar (up or down) can lead to fluctuations in inflammatory balance and thus in free-radical load. Higher levels of glucose in the blood lead to glycation of proteins (attachment of sugar molecules to the protein), including the proteins collagen, keratin, and elastin, which form part of the skin. Glycated molecules tend to be dysfunctional; glycated collagen molecules have reduced strength and break down faster, while glycated elastin fibers lose much of their elasticity. As a result, skin sags, wrinkles, and loses its snap. And if all that weren't bad enough, we also know that stress, and its primary hormone, cortisol, can lead to higher blood-sugar levels (thereby increasing glycation) and higher levels of inflammation (thereby setting off a chain reaction between eicosanoids and free radicals). All this leads to greater levels of oxidative damage to cells throughout the body—including in the skin.

CONTROLLING THE DAMAGE WITH THE "FACE" PROGRAM

Sounds pretty serious, doesn't it? But there is a way out—and by now, you probably have more than a glimmer of what it is. It's the FACE program, which you can use with terrific results to modulate every one of these metabolic factors to fully address the overall aging process. What follows is a discussion of the kinds of damage these factors can produce, along with a brief mention of FACE solutions. (You will find descriptions of these recommendations in much greater detail in subsequent chapters.)

F = Free Radicals

The Damage: Free radicals lead to oxidation (damage) of cellular membranes and DNA. Oxidized cells do not perform optimally and can lead to disease and dysfunction in all tissues —including the skin. Free radicals are directly associated with wrinkles and with elevated levels of inflammation (eicosanoids; see below), which leads to further tissue damage.

The Control: Free radicals can be controlled by antioxidants, such as vitamin C, vitamin E, alpha-lipoic acid, flavonoids (as in grape seed, green tea, citrus, and others), and carotenoids (such as beta-carotene, lycopene, lutein, and others). Antioxidants can be found in brightly colored fruits and vegetables, as well as in dietary supplements.

A = Age-Related Glycation End-Products (AGEs)

The Damage: AGEs are the result of proteins being exposed to elevated levels of blood sugar. Glycated proteins have impaired function and are broken down faster, leading to weakened tissue strength. In the case of skin, this means delayed wound healing, loss of elasticity, dehydration/dryness, and an overall loss of smoothness. Elevated blood sugar also leads directly to increased inflammatory load (more eicosanoids; see below) and increased free-radical damage.

The Control: AGEs can be controlled by eating fewer processed foods and more whole foods (to maintain normal blood glucose), as well as by using certain glucose-control supplements, such as alpha-lipoic acid (also an antioxidant), banaba leaf, gymnema, fenugreek, and others.

C = Cortisol

The Damage: Cortisol is the primary stress hormone. Cortisol overexposure leads directly and rapidly to elevated blood sugar (increasing glycation), as well as increased levels of free radicals and eicosanoids. Of the four metabolic factors addressed by FACE, cortisol control can be thought of as "first in line" because it so strongly influences the direction of the other three and because it serves as a signal in the body for the rapid breakdown of collagen (the chief structural protein in skin). Cortisol is also one of the primary causes of skin redness, rosacea, and oil overproduction (leading to acne), so controlling cortisol effectively yields skin benefits beyond the simple slowing of the aging process.

The Control: That said, a truly comprehensive skin-health regimen will build on cortisol control by modulating the remaining three areas of metabolism simultaneously. Cortisol can be controlled by exercise, yoga, stress management, balancing protein/fat/carb intake, and by a variety of antistress supplements, including theanine, magnolia bark, beta-sitosterol, phosphatidylserine, omega-3 fatty acids (also an anti-inflammatory), cordyceps, ginseng, ashwagandha, rhodiola, and others.

E = Eicosanoids

The Damage: Sometimes referred to as cytokines, eicosanoids are hormonelike compounds produced by cells to communicate with one another. The immune system is the primary source of eicosanoids, with both inflammatory and anti-inflammatory forms existing in the body at all times. The problem with eicosanoids is not that they are "bad," but rather that having too many of the inflammatory type and too few of the anti-inflammatory type leads directly to tissue damage, as well as to higher levels of both free radicals (and the destruction they cause) and cortisol overexposure (leading to glycation and the resulting tissue damage).

The Control: Eicosanoids can be controlled by limiting intake of inflammatory fatty acids (such as omega-6 fatty acids, found in most vegetable oils) and increasing intake of anti-inflammatory fatty acids (such as omega-3 fatty acids, found in fatty fish and fish oil supplements). Omega-3 fatty acids can also help to control cortisol levels.

The interrelations between each of these areas of metabolism means that affecting one area in a positive direction generally has a positive effect on the other three areas. *Even better, however, is to employ simple strategies to balance all four areas simultaneously.* For example, the development (or prevention) of wrinkles is strongly linked to imbalances in all four areas—

1. Free radicals (microdamage to the skin)

2. AGEs (loss of elastin function)

3. Cortisol (accelerated collagen breakdown)

4. Eicosanoids (inflammatory damage and free-radical promotion)

—so the full FACE program can work wonders here.

A BRIEF NOTE ON FACE
AND SPECIFIC SKIN CONDITIONS

Different skin conditions tend to be affected more by certain areas needing control. Although acne, for example, has a theoretical and biochemical association with free radicals and AGEs, it is linked more dramatically with cortisol (oil overproduction) and eicosanoids (inflammation). Both dry and oily skin are tightly linked to cortisol (accelerated collagen breakdown in the case of dry skin and oil overproduction in the case of oily skin), but individual differences in free-radical balance and AGE exposure will tip the scales toward a drier or oilier skin type from one person to the next. Skin redness and uneven skin tone can certainly be influenced by stress and cortisol levels, but the primary drivers here are free radicals (skin microdamage) and eicosanoids (inflammation). Skin that heals slowly would also benefit from the full FACE program, but especially from modulation of cortisol (accelerated collagen breakdown, suppressed immune response) and AGEs (poor circulation).

LIFESTYLE FACTORS THAT
CONTRIBUTE TO THE AGING PROCESS

Like other bodily systems, skin health is affected by our lifestyle choices. For example, one recent study investigating the impact of stress on wound healing in healthy nonsmoking men found that as stress increased, so did the amount of time it took for skin wounds to heal. Researchers determined that elevated cortisol levels were most likely to blame.

Tobacco consumption is hazardous to your health in a variety of ways, including skin damage. A single cigarette contains more than one hundred trillion free radicals, so each puff delivers a potent dose of cell-destroying oxidation to your delicate skin. A review study conducted by German researchers reported the following detrimental effects of smoking on skin health: (1) weakened collagen production that results in impaired wound healing and premature skin aging; (2) a heightened inflammatory response that plays a role in many skin diseases, such as psoriasis, atopic dermatitis, and acne; and (3) suppression of the immune system, which may contribute to malignant melanoma and epithelial skin tumors.

According to experts at the Cleveland Clinic, sun exposure is what causes most of the skin changes we think of as normal aspects of aging, such as loss of elasticity, mottled pigmentation, benign tumors, and fine and coarse wrinkles. But it's the connection between sun exposure and skin cancer that's the greatest reason for concern. Ultraviolet radiation from the sun is the number-one cause of several types of skin cancer, including basal cell and squamous cell carcinomas, as well as the more deadly form called melanoma. Cleveland Clinic experts say that cumulative sun exposure (and the cycle of oxidation/inflammation that results) is the main culprit for basal cell and squamous cell skin cancer, while severe sunburns in younger years can cause melanoma later in life.

Research continues to uncover more information, but scientists have already found many factors that contribute to the aging process. For example, skin cells divide more slowly with advancing years, and the inner dermal layer thins. This thinning network of elastin and collagen is less able to support the outer epidermis, and skin begins to form lines and to sag. Oil-secreting glands are less efficient and skin retains less moisture with age, contributing to the formation of wrinkles.

Fortunately, there's plenty you can do to fend off these challenges. Your skin regenerates itself approximately every twenty-seven days, which means that every month you've got a new opportunity to infuse this crucial organ with radiance and vitality. Drinking plenty of water, thorough cleansing and moisturizing, consistent use of a full-spectrum sunscreen (one that blocks both UVA and UVB rays), wholesome nutrition, regular exercise, a few key supplements, and a healthy lifestyle are all factors that add up to total skin wellness. Some evidence even suggests that massage may support a healthy glow.

SUPPORTING NUTRIENTS
GIVING COLLAGEN A HELPING HAND

It makes very little sense for anybody to talk about nutrition or dietary supplementation without putting it into the context of how it can help the entire body. I can tell you that calcium is good for your bones, but without considering your intake of other nutrients, such as vitamin D, magnesium, phosphorous, protein, and sodium, a recommendation to "get more calcium" is little more than a shot in the dark. The same goes for dietary supplements intended to support skin metabolism.

The process by which amino acids are used by the body to produce healthy collagen fibers is a complicated one. Along the way, a number of specialized enzymes and active cofactors must be present in just the right amounts and at just the right times for the whole process to operate optimally. Among these active cofactors are vitamins C, D, E, and B complex, as well as the minerals copper, zinc, manganese, and silicon, which are vital components of the collagen-production machinery. In addition, there is a wide variety of non-nutrient factors, such as bromelain, boswellia, green tea, grape seed, and gotu kola, that may be able to enhance the process of connective-tissue maintenance by reducing inflammation and improving circulation.

In the forthcoming chapters, you'll learn about the most effective ingredients to support healthy skin from the inside. For now, let's take a brief look at some of the fundamental ways in which nutritional habits affect collagen health.

Glycation Control

Scientists now know that microinflammation (inflammation on a scale too small to be seen) in the skin can be caused by excessive exposure to both free radicals and glycation, each of which leads to its own form of accelerated aging. Some of the main dietary offenders in this cycle are high-sugar foods such as candy, ice cream, donuts, cookies, and sugary breakfast cereals, as well as other foods with a high glycemic index, for example, processed grains such as those found in white bread, white rolls, or instant rice. (A food with a high glycemic index is one that quickly converts to sugar or glucose in the bloodstream.) Sugar can be toxic to your skin when it permanently attaches to collagen fibers through the glycation process. Wherever sugar attaches, it triggers a biochemical mechanism that creates inflammation. The inflammation, in turn, produces enzymes that break down collagen, thus resulting in wrinkles. To make matters worse, glycation also leads to the cross-linking of collagen fibers, changing skin from soft and supple to stiff and brittle. These stiff sugar-protein bonds form in other tissues too, such as veins, arteries, tendons, and ligaments—which is why some scientists are now finding links between glycation and cardiovascular disease or arthritis.

Over the Rainbow

In a nutshell, then, high-glycemic/high-sugar/highly processed foods flood the body with sugar (glucose), which then wreaks havoc on skin collagen. So that's what *not* to eat. But what foods can *promote* skin health?

Start by looking for the rainbow—of vividly colored foods, that is. Plant pigments don't just make foods pretty; they also make them potently nutritious. In addition to being great sources of vitamins A and C—necessary nutrients for skin maintenance and repair—colorful foods also contain phytonutrients (*phyto* means "plant"), which contain numerous disease-preventing, anti-inflammatory, antiaging antioxidants.

The free radical–fighting antioxidants found in colorful foods provide broad skin-health benefits, such as reducing inflammation by neutralizing free radicals produced during the inflammatory process. And some exert other effects, such as strengthening the vascular system, blocking sun damage, and directly preventing glycation. A special group of these antioxidants called flavonoids exerts strong anti-inflammatory effects by inhibiting certain cyclooxygenase (COX) enzymes. COX-1 enzymes are the good guys, acting to protect the stomach and intestinal lining. COX-2 enzymes, on the other hand, are the ones that cause pain and inflammation. Nonsteroidal anti-inflammatory drugs (NSAIDs), such as aspirin and ibuprofen, block both groups of COX enzymes, which is why they're effective at reducing pain and inflammation yet carry the potential side effect of stomach and intestinal erosion. However, flavonoids, such as those found in ginger, grape seed extract, turmeric, and other herbs and spices, are able to block primarily the inflammatory COX-2 enzymes, thereby reducing inflammation without the toxic side effects.

The richer the color of a food, the better: Deep color indicates a greater concentration of these antioxidants. Since different colors represent different antioxidant nutrients, select from as many different-colored foods as possible, including fruits (apples, blueberries, blackberries, strawberries, raspberries, oranges, mangoes, kiwifruit, tomatoes), vegetables (spinach, green bell peppers, eggplant, red bell peppers, pumpkin, squash, corn, yams, onions), and brown-toned nuts, seeds, and legumes. A good rule of thumb is to include multicolored foods with every meal and snack—at least one serving, or about a half cup.

Good Fats

In the last few years, considerable media attention has been paid to delineating between bad fats and good ones. The now-golden rule of reducing bad fats, such as saturated fats (e.g., those contained in whole-milk dairy products and fatty red meat and poultry) and trans-fats (hydrogenated and partially hydrogenated oils), applies to skin health too—as long as you also include the good guys: essential fatty acids (EFAs). Research has shown that EFAs—in particular, omega-3 fatty acids—afford healing benefits in various inflammatory conditions, such as rheumatoid arthritis and skin eczema, and that they may exert their anti-inflammatory effects by blocking COX-2 enzymes. Omega-3s are also effective controllers of cortisol overexposure and, as such, can help keep skin supple and guard against wrinkle formation.

Fatty acids are the building blocks of all fats, but the ones termed "essential" are so named because, like essential amino acids and vitamins and minerals, your body cannot produce them. You must get these health-promoting fats from outside sources. The average American gets plenty of one type of EFA —omega-6 fats (linoleic acid). Cutting back on your intake of vegetable oils high in linolenic acid, such as safflower oil, sunflower oil, and corn oil, is one way to reduce your intake of pro-inflammatory omega-6 fats. Yet our diets are often lacking in omega-3 fats (linolenic acid), such as eicosapentaenoic acid (EPA) and docosahexaenoic acid (DHA). Good food sources of omega-3s include fatty fish, such as salmon, tuna, mackerel, herring, and sardines, along with ground flaxseed, flaxseed oil, canola oil, and walnuts. Some skin-health experts suggest including a source of EFAs with every meal, while other researchers say several times a week is enough. Fish and flaxseed oil are also available in supplement form at most health food stores.

Don't Forget the H_2O

The amount of water you need to properly hydrate skin and move nutrients in and toxins out varies with several factors, including environmental conditions and your activity level (both of which affect how much fluid you lose as sweat). Experts, however, generally suggest an intake reminiscent of the old standby: eight to ten glasses a day (a "glass" consists of eight fluid ounces, i.e., one cup, or about eight good-sized swallows). Any good, clean water works, but the National Academy of Sciences states that hard water—the kind high in minerals—may be even better for health, due to the higher level of nutrients, such as calcium and magnesium, it contains.

EXERCISE YOUR SKIN

When the subject is exercise, you probably think of weight loss, toned muscles, strong bones, and a healthy heart, but you may not think about how exercise benefits your skin. Yet experts say that regular exercise can influence skin health in many ways. For example, it's well known that exercise enhances circulation, and along with better circulation goes better nutrient delivery to skin cells, as well as more efficient toxin removal. Additionally, plenty of evidence says that exercise reduces stress, which, in turn, calms the adrenal glands. Calmer adrenals mean a lower production of testosterone-related hormones, such as dehydroepiandrosterone (DHEA) and dihydrotestosterone (DHT), which are often implicated in acne flare-ups. It follows, then, that exercise specifically directed at mind-body stress reduction, such as yoga, tai chi, and qi gong, may have a particularly beneficial effect on acne-prone skin. Another consideration: These same stress-reducing types of exercise support total-body relaxation, including relaxation of the muscles in your face, which, some experts say, softens expression lines.

But just about any kind of exercise can be beneficial for your skin if you consider that sweating improves skin health. The thinking goes that sweating opens and unclogs pores, which has a positive effect on skin breakouts. So anything that encourages sweating could help clear up acne.

Just as exercise turns back the clock for muscles and bones, it may also afford antiaging effects for your skin. With advancing years, not only do our bodies have fewer fibroblasts (the skin's collagen-producing cells), but the ones we do have aren't quite as ambitious as they once were. As a result, skin sags and wrinkles. But jazz up your skin-care routine with exercise, and the resulting enhanced circulation brings more oxygen and other nutrients to cells, thereby creating an ideal environment for ramped-up collagen production. Increased circulation will help deliver vital nutrients through the blood to the dermis and eventually to the surface epidermis, the layer of skin that can be seen. The easy-to-follow exercise program outlined in Appendix B shows you how to use physical activity to increase systemic circulation.

One more thing: Remember the earlier discussion of the connection between sugar, glycation, and skin aging? Since exercise stabilizes blood sugar, it could, in theory, reduce the potential for glycation's inflammatory aging effects.

A CONCLUDING WORD

There are vast amounts of scientific and medical information concerning the details underlying each of the metabolic processes I discuss in this book—far too much info to even summarize here. For interested readers, I invite you to more fully explore these intricacies at my Cortisol Connection website (www.cortisolconnection.com) and also the controlling/modulating role played by specific nutrients at my Supplement Watch website (www.supplementwatch.com). Both sites are updated routinely—much faster than what can be accomplished with printed media. By visiting these websites, you can gain a greater understanding of the role each area plays in skin health and how you can tap into them to create your own fountain of youth.

CHAPTER 4

. . . .
.
.

Inside–Out Help for Wrinkles, Acne, and "Problem" Skin

Beauty is how you feel inside, and it reflects in your eyes.
It is not something physical.

— Sophia Loren, Italian actress

A popular antiwrinkle book identifies free radicals as "the cause" of wrinkles and antioxidant creams as "the cure" for wrinkles. Another "face-lift" book identifies inflammation as "the cause" of premature aging and a daily diet of salmon as "the cure" for aging skin (in the two-week program, you'd be eating fish thirty-one times in fourteen days). Yet another anti-acne book argues that all you need to do to prevent and treat pimples is to buy the author's line of expensive creams and lotions.

What each of these popular books misses, however, is the complex nature of our metabolic machinery. By now, you should be well aware that skin "problems," such as wrinkles, acne, redness, rosacea, and others, are caused by a much more complex series of events than the single "villains" named in many popular books. As you now know, it's the interplay between at least four areas of metabolism (and perhaps more that we do not yet fully understand) that predisposes all of us to having certain types of skin problems now and other types a few months from now.

If you look at Figure 4.1, you'll quickly notice that cortisol (C) exposure leads to increases in free radicals (F), advanced glycation (A), and eicosanoids (E). Likewise, an increase in free radicals (F) leads in turn to an increase in eicosanoids (E) and vice versa. This back-and-forth interplay continues unabated if you focus on controlling a single area (such as free radicals) without also considering the other areas (such as cortisol).

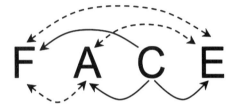

Figure 4.1: The complex interplay among the metabolic factors that contribute to aging skin (solid lines represent one-way influences; dotted lines represent two-way interactions)

Luckily, a coordinated approach to controlling all four of these metabolic pathways is not difficult. By following the Helping Hand approach to eating (as outlined in Chapter 5) and incorporating some of the recipes from Appendix A into your diet, you can do a great deal to rebalance each of these pathways.

WRINKLES

We know that the development of wrinkles is related to *each* of the four aspects of metabolism addressed by FACE, as well as by a gradual loss of water (dehydration) from the skin. As collagen and elastin fibers in healthy skin are damaged by overexposure to free radicals, advanced glycation, cortisol, and eicosanoids, they lose their ability to regenerate themselves, causing the skin to wrinkle.

The "solution," then, to reversing existing wrinkles and preventing new wrinkles from developing becomes a battle to control these aspects of metabolism. Follow the dietary advice spelled out in Part II of the book. In addition, virtually any exercise regimen or activity that you enjoy will help to increase blood circulation to the skin, which will enhance delivery of nutrients and removal of waste products.

ACNE

The skin condition called "acne" is due to a disorder of the oil glands, which results in clogged pores and outbreaks of lesions commonly known as pimples. Acne is the most common skin disease in the U.S., affecting between seventeen million and forty-five million people, male and female. Acne is most common in adolescence, and although it usually disappears by around age thirty, in its severe state it can cause pain and permanent scarring, both physical and emotional. Sometimes acne occurs, or recurs, in women well into middle age.

It is thought that acne may be caused or worsened by such factors as a family history of acne; greasy/oily cosmetic or hair products containing vegetable or animal fats; hormonal changes associated with adolescence, pregnancy, menstruation, or premenopause; certain medications; environmental irritants such as industrial cutting oils, tar, wood preservatives, sealing compounds, and other pollutants; high levels of humidity; oily sunscreens; and, not surprisingly, stress.

We know that acne is caused by a step-by-step process, starting with clogged pores, overproduction of oil, and bacterial growth leading to inflammation. *The clogging of pores is not (as is commonly believed) caused by "dirty" skin, but rather by an overgrowth of keratin, the hard collagen-derived protein forming the outermost layer of skin*. Once the pore becomes blocked, the stage is set for a cortisol/stress-induced overproduction of oil. I'm sure you've noticed that you have more breakouts when you're under the most stress. The cause of those extra pimples is cortisol stimulating an increase in oil production in the skin. Next, the bacteria that naturally occur on your skin get trapped in that excess oil, where they break down the oil molecules, leading to an inflammatory response (and the associated pain and redness of a pimple).

If we break this process down into its root biochemical causes, we see that each of the imbalances in the chain of events leading to a pimple can be wonderfully modified by FACE. From disrupted keratin/collagen metabolism, to cortisol exposure and oil overproduction, to inflammation—all are central to the FACE program.

ROSACEA, ECZEMA, DERMATITIS— AND OTHER JOYS

Studies suggest that close to fifty million Americans are affected by one or more of these very common skin conditions. It is interesting to note that each has a root biochemical cause related to inflammation and stress. Although the precise "triggering event" may vary from person to person, stress and inflammation are hallmarks of rosacea, eczema, and dermatitis. As such, regimens that control these aspects of metabolism can do wonders for the red, itchy patches that often appear without warning.

Eczema, which is a form of dermatitis, is a chronic, inflammatory skin disorder, most often resulting in blisters that dry into scaly, itchy rashes. As moisture is lost from the skin's upper layer, it becomes dry and itchy, leaving the skin without protection and thus inviting bacteria and viruses to penetrate. Sometimes the symptoms are severe (flares) and sometimes there are no symptoms at all (remission). Eczema is not contagious. People with eczema often have a personal or family history of allergic conditions, such as asthma or hay fever. Exposure to irritants and allergens in the environment can worsen symptoms—for example, certain soaps, detergents, perfumes, and cosmetics; wool or synthetic fibers; certain metals, such as nickel; and cigarette smoke. So can stress, dry skin, exposure to water, and changes in temperature. Although there is no cure, there are ways to reduce symptoms and help prevent outbreaks.

WHY IS CORTISOL CONTROL SO IMPORTANT?

As you'll notice from the FACE diagram above, stress and cortisol exposure can set off higher levels of inflammation (E = eicosanoids), oxidation (F = free radicals), and glycation (A = advanced glycation end-products, AGEs). Numerous studies of cortisol and its effects on skin have shown that cortisol overexposure (from emotional stress or sleep deprivation) can

- increase oil production in the skin (leading to acne)
- increase appetite for sweets (leading to glycation, collagen breakdown, and wrinkles)
- interfere with insulin function (increasing blood-sugar levels and glycation)
- increase eicosanoids and related cytokines (leading to reduced wound healing, slower skin regeneration, and more redness/itchiness/swelling)
- increase free-radical load (leading to skin microdamage and loss of moisture and barrier protection)

Interestingly, the "stress" of exercise does *not* lead to a similar list of skin complaints; instead, it can actually alleviate a range of skin problems. For example, although moderate exercise leads to a temporary elevation in cortisol levels and free-radical exposure, the body's cortisol and free-radical levels for the rest of the day are much lower. This is one of the significant antistress benefits of regular exercise. In addition, exercise—or any type of regular physical activity—leads to positive metabolic changes that are good for the skin, including the following:

- Increased circulation, delivery of nutrients, and removal of wastes to/from the skin

- Increased insulin sensitivity (leading to lower blood sugar and reduced glycation)

- Improved antioxidant defenses (leading to reduced oxidative damage in all parts of the body, including the skin

- Reduced eicosanoid load (leading to lower levels of systemic inflammation, which is good for the heart, brain, and skin)

Because of the wide-ranging influence that cortisol has on other important aspects of metabolism—especially the metabolic pathways associated most closely with "aging"—as mentioned earlier, cortisol is often called the "death hormone." This nickname is apropos because cortisol is one of only two hormones that tend to increase with age. (The other is insulin; however, a large part of the insulin rise can be controlled by modulating cortisol levels.) This gradual increase in cortisol exposure as we age has been linked to breakdown and dysfunction in every tissue of the body. So whether we're talking about skin or heart muscle or brain neurons, it makes sense to address cortisol as sort of a "master switch" in aging metabolism.

This is not to say that cortisol is the only metabolic pathway that needs to be controlled in order to promote healthy skin. Rather, cortisol control is the most logical place to start, using a truly comprehensive program that simultaneously addresses each of the other aspects of FACE (the oxidation, glycation, and inflammation that result when they're uncontrolled).

A CONCLUDING WORD

This chapter explained the key aspects of the metabolism underlying the development of wrinkles, acne, rosacea, and other skin problems. You will learn more about these conditions—and what to do to help treat them—in Chapter 11.

Now we move to Part II of the book, where you will be given specific tools for dealing with your own skin. In Chapters 5 through 9, you will find specific advice on diet and on nutritional supplements that are known to be effective in addressing each of the four FACE metabolic pathways. In Chapter 10, you will receive a weekly step-by-step guide to starting and following the FACE program to help you take control of your skin and your health. And in Chapter 11, you will see what several skin-care experts suggest about caring for that most important and sensitive organ, your skin.

PART II

Tools to *Beautify* Your Skin

CHAPTER 5

. . . .
.
.

Good Taste Equals
Good Looks:
How Nutrition Can
Support Beautiful Skin

In writing the original book in this series, *The Cortisol Connection: Why Stress Makes You Fat and Ruins Your Health—and What You Can Do About It* (2002), and the follow-up book, *The Cortisol Connection Diet: The Breakthrough Program to Control Stress and Lose Weight* (2004), and after conducting dozens of cortisol-control programs (mostly geared toward weight loss) for hundreds of participants, something dawned on me and my research staff in sort of a collective "lightbulb" moment: We realized that the lifestyle regimen for cortisol control is the same as the regimen for weight loss and for skin health and for mental functioning and for energy levels…and on and on.

Whenever we looked at a chronic health condition and investigated its metabolic underpinnings, we found the same dysfunction and imbalance between the "usual suspects": those aspects of metabolism primarily related to cortisol, oxidation, inflammation, and glycation.

At first, we were perplexed—after all, how could a single regimen (even as multifaceted as it was) change the course of such a range of disparate diseases across every single organ system? The reason, we would eventually discover, is because in controlling and rebalancing these primary metabolic pathways, we were uncovering the very root of many modern disease processes, which are merely metabolic imbalances left unchecked.

These realizations provided us with some satisfaction (because we were helping hundreds of thousands of readers get to the root of their chronic conditions), but they also left us with a sense of unease—primarily that we might be missing something that could help people even more—and that's where dietary supplements and other natural products come in.

Although the general diet and exercise regimens you'll find in this book are essentially the same as the ones you'll find in *The Cortisol Connection Diet*, the supplement regimen outlined here is specifically tailored to support the unique metabolism of the skin. For example, two people could be following the same diet/exercise regimen to control cortisol, oxidation, inflammation, and glycation, but differences in their dietary supplement regimens will provide the tipping point to emphasize weight loss benefits for one person and anti-acne effects for the other.

Some readers may view this admission as a cop-out. They'll say, "Hey, this is the same weight loss diet I've already read about." While others, such as the hundreds of satisfied participants who have tried our diets, will instead say, "Terrific! I already know that this diet helps me lose weight and control my appetite. Now I know it can make me look better, think better, and feel better." What could be better than that?

If you're not convinced that a single way of eating can offer so many different benefits, then I invite you to give it a try. You have nothing to lose except your flab, your wrinkles, your pimples, your depression, and your fatigue.

THE HELPING HAND DIET

The eating strategy that the clients in our cortisol and weight programs follow is not about adhering to a strict meal-planning regimen; nor is it about restricting any foods or categories of foods. In fact, it's not much of a "diet" at all. Most of the people who have tried it can confirm that they often eat *more* food while following our advice—and they still lose weight. We call the diet the "Helping Hand" approach because you use the size of your hand as a portion-control device. This easy-to-follow plan teaches you how to balance your intake of carbohydrates, protein, fat, and fiber in a way that considers both the *quantity* of food and, even more importantly, the *quality* of those foods.

A simplified version of the Helping Hand diet is outlined below. For a more thorough description, please refer to my earlier book *The Cortisol Connection Diet* or to the Cortisol Connection website (www.cortisolconnection.com).

Quality: What to Eat
Step 1—Consider Carbohydrates
General rule: Foods that are more "whole" (in their natural, unprocessed state) are better for long-term control of oxidation, inflammation, glycation, and cortisol. Carbohydrates, in and of themselves, are not "bad," but the form of carbohydrate that you choose to consume will determine your body's metabolic response and your likelihood of storing that food as fat. Whenever possible, choose whole-grain bread and cereal products and fresh fruits and vegetables over their more processed counterparts.

Step 2—Provide Protein
General rule: Any form of lean protein can be used to "rebalance" a refined carbohydrate. Protein and carbs are the "yin and yang" of nutrition: They have to be consumed together

for proper dietary balance (which falls apart when either one is excluded or inappropriately restricted).

Step 3—Finish with Fat
General rule: A small amount of added fat at each meal is a "metabolic regulator." A bit of added fat—in the form of a pat of butter, a dash of olive oil, a square of cheese, or a handful of nuts—helps to slow the postmeal rise in blood sugar, which in turn helps to control appetite and enhance fat burning throughout the day.

Step 4—Fill Up with Fiber
General rule: Choosing "whole" forms of grains, fruits, and vegetables (as recommended in Step 1) will automatically satisfy your fiber needs. Like fat, fiber helps to slow the absorption of sugar from the digestive tract into the bloodstream. In this way, fiber can also be considered a "metabolic regulator" to help balance blood-sugar levels at each meal or snack.

Quantity: How Much to Eat
Use the following graphic depictions to determine appropriate serving sizes of each food group:

 Fruits and veggies: A serving = the size of your entire open hand

 Concentrated carbs (breads, potatoes, pasta, cereal, etc.): A serving = the size of your tightly closed fist

 Lean protein: A serving = the size of your palm

 Added fat: A serving = the size of the space created when you make an "okay" sign

This approach to eating considers both the quality and the quantity of every meal and snack—and the best part is that it requires *zero* counting of calories, fat grams, or carb grams. Why? Because the calorie control is already built in based on the size of your hands (Mother Nature's automatic portion control). A person with average-sized hands will consume about five hundred calories from each meal built using the Helping Hand approach.

Two Food Additives to Avoid

I'm not really a fan of the highly restrictive popular diets that cut out almost all carbs or most of the fat from your diet. These diets have poor long-term success rates and they're simply miserable to follow. For this reason, I don't like to tell people that there is any such thing as a "forbidden food" or a "banned list" of foods—but I make an exception for two food additives because of their extreme toxicity to the body and the dramatic metabolic disruption they trigger in all four of the FACE factors. These ingredients are high-fructose corn syrup and hydrogenated or partially hydrogenated oils.

High-Fructose Corn Syrup

High-fructose corn syrup (HFCS) is a sweetener made from corn. It is higher in fructose (the main sugar found in fruit) than regular corn syrup or table sugar, which is technically known as sucrose. The food industry likes to use HFCS because it is both cheaper and sweeter than regular sugar, so food manufacturers can use smaller amounts of it and save money compared to using pure sugar in order to sweeten processed foods. However, because fructose is metabolized quite differently from other sugars, overconsumption can result in some very dramatic alterations in energy metabolism—including disrupted cortisol metabolism, insulin resistance (leading to advanced glycation), and higher levels of systemic inflammation.

Hydrogenated Oils

Hydrogenated oils are liquid vegetable oils that have been chemically modified by pumping extra hydrogen atoms into their chemical structure to produce a solid or semisolid form—think Crisco or other vegetable shortenings. These hydrogenated oils, also called partially hydrogenated oils, trans-fats, or trans-fatty acids (which refers to the change in their chemical structure), are easier to handle than liquid oils during food processing, and they are preferred in many processed foods because they can add crispiness to crackers and longer shelf life to cookies. Trans-fats are known to interfere with the metabolism of cortisol (increasing cortisol levels), blood sugar (increasing blood glucose and inhibiting insulin function), and the inflammatory cascade (nudging it toward a proinflammatory state, which further interferes with cortisol metabolism).

The bad news is that both trans-fats and HFCS are found in high amounts in many processed foods. As a general rule of thumb, any food that lists either of these additives as one of the first three ingredients should automatically be considered off-limits in your quest to look and feel better.

Timing: When to Eat

The approach that we have found to be most effective represents a subtle but important departure from many popular diets. Like many existing programs, the Helping Hand plan encourages you to eat several small meals and snacks throughout the course of the day. This approach to eating can do wonders for modulating your blood sugar and cortisol responses to food, thereby helping to control appetite, boost energy levels, and encourage fat burning throughout the day—not to mention reducing the damaging effects of glycation and cortisol exposure on your skin.

The Helping Hand diet optimizes this approach by spacing three meals and three snacks throughout the day in the following pattern:

7:00 A.M.:   Snack (before leaving for work)

9:00 A.M.:   Breakfast (at work)

Noon: Snack (plus exercise if you can fit it in)

2:00 P.M.:   Lunch

5:00 P.M.:   Snack (before leaving work or on the way home)

7:00 P.M.:   Dinner (with a cocktail or a small dessert as your optional fourth "snack" of the day)

A snack consists of one appropriately sized serving from the fruit/veggie group, plus one appropriately sized serving of fat (such as some nuts and a piece of cheese). A meal consists of one appropriately sized serving from each of the starch, protein, and fat groups, plus one or two appropriately sized servings from the fruit/veggie group.

A CONCLUDING WORD

That's it. At this point, you can see how the Helping Hand approach to eating can be easy to follow, practical to use in your everyday life, and effective as a way to control the key aspects of metabolism related to the majority of chronic conditions facing us today.

The next four chapters explore some of the options available for dietary supplements to fine-tune this baseline metabolic control toward wrinkle reduction, acne alleviation, or simply balancing of skin tone by controlling cortisol, free radicals, glycation, and inflammation.

. . . .
                    .
                    .

CHAPTER 6

Supplements for the Control of Cortisol

Even though cortisol comes third in the FACE acronym, it really is of primary importance because of its intimate interactions with the other three aspects of FACE (refer to the FACE diagram in Chapter 4). As such, we'll consider supplements for cortisol control first. Keep in mind that many of the supplements that are effective primarily for cortisol control are also effective as secondary controllers of blood sugar (and thus glycation), free radicals (and thus oxidation), and eicosanoids/cytokines (and thus inflammation).

The science regarding dietary supplements and nutrition changes rapidly, so I encourage you to visit my website www .cortisolconnection.com for frequent updates on dietary regimens and other lifestyle strategies for controlling the myriad aspects of metabolism associated with skin health.

BETA-SITOSTEROL

Beta-sitosterol is one of hundreds of plant-derived "sterol" compounds that are known to influence cortisol exposure, immune function, and inflammation. Plant oils contain the highest concentration of phytosterols, so nuts and seeds contain fairly high levels and all fruits and vegetables generally contain some amount. Perhaps the best way to obtain beta-sitosterol is to eat a diet rich in fruits, vegetables, nuts, and seeds (which obviously brings numerous other benefits, too), but beta-sitosterol is available in supplement form as well.

Beta-sitosterol is known to modulate immune function, inflammation, and pain levels through its effects on controlling the production of inflammatory cytokines. Much of this immune/inflammation control appears to be related to an improved interaction of immune cells (which produce eicosanoids and cytokines) with the adrenal glands (which produce cortisol). This modulation of cytokine production and activity may help control allergic skin reactions such as rosacea, dermatitis, and eczema, while also helping to promote general skin-barrier function and wound healing.

In terms of immune function, beta-sitosterol has been shown in humans to normalize the function of T-helper lymphocytes and natural killer cells following stressful events (such as marathon running) that normally suppress immune-system function. In addition to alleviating much of the post-exercise immune suppression that occurs following endurance competitions, beta-sitosterol has also been shown to normalize the ratio of catabolic stress hormones (cortisol) to anabolic (rebuilding) hormones such as DHEA.

No significant side effects or drug interactions have been reported in any of the studies investigating beta-sitosterol, and the widespread presence of beta-sitosterol in the diet means that it is generally recognized as an extremely safe supplement with no side effects.

The typical daily dosage of beta-sitosterol for immune-function and cortisol-controlling benefits is 60–120 mg. A handful of roasted peanuts or a couple of tablespoons of peanut butter will contain about 10–30 mg of beta-sitosterol.

ASHWAGANDHA *(WITHANIA SOMNIFERA)*

Ashwagandha is an herb native to India that is sometimes called winter cherry or "Indian ginseng"—to suggest energy-promoting and antistress benefits similar to those attributed to the better-known Asian and Siberian ginsengs. Herbalists and natural-medicine practitioners often recommend ashwagandha to help combat stress and fatigue. In traditional Indian (Ayurvedic) medicine, ashwagandha is used to "balance life forces" during stress and aging.

Because of its relaxation and general antistress benefits, ashwagandha is commonly used to enhance mental and physical performance, improve learning ability and mental function, decrease stress, and relieve insomnia.

Most of what we know about ashwagandha comes from reports of traditional use in humans by practitioners of Ayurvedic medicine and from experimental studies in animals. In the animal studies, ashwagandha has shown benefits in treating both anxiety and depression, boosting immune-system function, enhancing the antitumor effects of chemotherapy, stimulating thyroid function, and improving memory and mental function. Many of these effects are likely due to a modulation of cortisol metabolism during periods of high stress. During stress, elevated cortisol levels can lead to depression, anxiety, a suppressed immune system, reduced thyroid function, and mental decline; ashwagandha may relieve some of the stress-induced elevation in cortisol levels and help return metabolism to normal.

In terms of safety, there are no reports of adverse side effects in humans, and acute toxicity studies in rodents have shown ashwagandha to have a wide margin of safety (in excess of 3,000 mg/day). Because of the effects of ashwagandha on muscle relaxation and as a mild central-nervous-system depressant, the herb should not be combined with alcohol or other sedatives, sleep aids, or anxiolytics (antianxiety medications). Pregnant women are advised to avoid ashwagandha due to its reported abortifacient (abortion-inducing) effects and potential for causing premature labor.

General dosage recommendations for ashwagandha are in the range of 200–800 mg per day of an extract standardized to 1–2 percent withanolides (the herb's primary active components).

CORDYCEPS *(CORDYCEPS SINENSIS)*

Cordyceps is a mushroom used in traditional Chinese medicine (TCM) for "invigoration" as well as to balance the chi—the fundamental energy of life. In some ways, cordyceps is a bit like ginseng in that both supplements are known to have effects on reducing stress, boosting stamina, and increasing energy levels. Both are also excellent controllers of blood-sugar levels. Although the pharmacologically active components of cordyceps remain unknown, at least two chemical constituents, cordycepin (deoxyadenosine) and cordycepic acid (mannitol), have been identified and suggested as being the active compounds in improving energy and stamina.

Animal studies have shown that feeding cordyceps can increase the ratio of adenosine triphosphate (ATP) to inorganic phosphate (Pi) in the liver by 45–55 percent—an effect that may be viewed as beneficial in terms of energy state and potential for performance enhancement. Furthermore, mice fed cordyceps and subjected to an extremely low oxygen environment were able to utilize oxygen more efficiently (30–50 percent increase), better tolerate acidosis and hypoxia (lack of oxygen), and live two to three times longer than a control group.

In a number of Chinese clinical studies, primarily of elderly patients suffering from fatigue, cordyceps-treated patients reported significant improvements in their level of fatigue, ability to tolerate cold temperatures, memory and cognitive capacity, and sex drive. Patients with respiratory diseases also reported feeling physically stronger. Recently, a small study presented at the annual meeting of the American College of

Sports Medicine showed that cordyceps significantly increases maximal oxygen uptake and anaerobic threshold, which may lead to improved exercise capacity and resistance to fatigue.

There are no known side effects associated with cordyceps, though effective daily dosages need to be in the range of 1–2 grams to deliver meaningful control of cortisol levels.

EPIMEDIUM

Epimedium is sometimes referred to as "horny goat weed" because of its traditional use in treating fatigue and boosting sex drive. The use of epimedium as a medicinal herb dates back to at least 400 A.D. It has been used as a tonic for the reproductive system (boosting libido and treating impotence) and for rejuvenation (to relieve fatigue and reduce stress). Epimedium is thought to work via modulation of cortisol levels. Under conditions of high stress, increased cortisol levels are known to cause fatigue and depress sex drive, so bringing cortisol levels back into normal ranges is thought to help restore normal metabolism, energy levels, and libido.

Animal studies have shown that epimedium may function a bit like an adaptogen (examples of which include cordyceps, rhodiola, ashwagandha, and ginseng) by increasing levels of epinephrine, norepinephrine, serotonin, and dopamine when they are low (an energy-promoting effect), but reducing cortisol levels when they are elevated (an antistress effect). There is also evidence that epimedium can restore low levels of both testosterone and thyroid hormone back to their normal levels, which may account for some of the benefits of epimedium in improving sex drive. Animal studies using epimedium have shown a reduction in bone breakdown, an increase in muscle mass, and a loss of body fat, each of which may be linked to the observed return of abnormal cortisol levels and rhythm back to normal. In a series of studies conducted in humans and animals by Chinese researchers, immune-system function was directly suppressed and bone loss was accelerated by using high-dose synthetic cortisol (glucocorticoid drugs). Subsequent administration of epimedium extract reduced blood levels of cortisol and improved immune-system function (in the humans) and slowed bone loss and strengthened bones (in the animals).

It is interesting to note that although at least fifteen active compounds have been identified in epimedium extracts (including luteolin, icariin, quercetin, and various epimedins), many supplement companies currently use alcohol extracts standardized only for high levels of icariin. The traditional way to use epimedium, however, is as a hot-water decoction (tea), which would result in a very different profile of active constituents when compared to the high-icariin alcohol extracts that are more commonly used in many commercial products. Although at least one test-tube study has shown icariin to protect liver cells from damage by various toxic compounds, other feeding studies (in rodents) have suggested that high-dose icariin may be associated with kidney and liver toxicity. There have been no reports of adverse side effects associated with the traditional preparation of epimedium (water-extracted) at the suggested dosage (250–1,000 mg per day).

DAMIANA

Damina leaves have been traditionally used as a respiratory, neurological, and sexual medicine by the indigenous cultures of Mexico. Damiana has also been used as an aphrodisiac and has been claimed to induce euphoria—both effects largely due to damiana's effects on controlling cortisol exposure.

Damiana's ability to induce mild euphoria could support a logical theory that in relatively small quantities, damiana could lead to relaxation and could calm anxiety, stress, and, thus, cortisol. Conceivably, those suffering from sexual dysfunction resulting from stress or emotional troubles could benefit from supplementation with this herb. Perhaps the most viable scientific evidence for the age-old use of damiana as an antistress supplement involves a recent study demonstrating that damiana extract mimics some of the actions of progesterone, suggesting that damiana could help alleviate some of the hormonal changes associated with menopause, such as high stress, increased cortisol levels, thinner skin and hair, and generalized skin problems. Likewise, damiana extract could ease the cyclical depression and anxiety often associated with women's menstrual cycles. That said, since the scientific community has not rigorously studied damiana, the herb is not recommended for women who are pregnant or lactating, for children, or for anyone with a serious medical condition or who is taking prescription medication.

General dosage recommendations call for 400–800 mg of damiana daily, but dosage recommendations may vary somewhat based on the combination of other ingredients in a particular product.

MAGNOLIA BARK *(MAGNOLIA OFFICINALIS)*

Magnolia bark, a traditional Chinese medicine known as *houpu* or *hou po*, has been used since 100 A.D. for treating "stagnation of chi" (low energy), as well as a variety of syndromes, such as digestive disturbances caused by emotional distress and turmoil. Modern-day use of magnolia bark is as a general antistress and antianxiety agent.

Magnolia bark is rich in two biphenol compounds, magnolol and honokiol, which are thought to contribute to the primary antistress and cortisol-lowering effects of the plant. The magnolol content of magnolia bark is generally in the range of 2–10 percent, while honokiol tends to occur naturally at 1–5 percent in dried magnolia bark. Magnolia bark also contains a bit less than 1 percent of an essential oil known as eudesmol, which is classified as a triterpene compound and may provide some additional benefits as an antioxidant.

Two of the most popular herbal medicines used in Japan, one called *Saiboku-to* and another called *Hange-kobuku-to*, contain magnolia bark and have been used for treating ailments from bronchial asthma to depression to anxiety. Japanese researchers have determined that the magnolol and honokiol components of *Magnolia officinalis* are one thousand times more potent than alpha-tocopherol (vitamin E) in their antioxidant activity, thereby offering a potential heart-health benefit. Other research groups have shown that both magnolol and honokiol possess powerful brain-health benefits via their actions in modulating the activity of various neurotransmitters and related enzymes in the brain (increased choline acetyltransferase activity, inhibition of acetylcholinesterase, and increased acetylcholine release). Numerous animal studies have demonstrated honokiol to act as a central-nervous-system depressant at high doses, but as a nonsedating anxiolytic (antianxiety and antistress) agent at lower doses. This means that a small dose of honokiol, or a magnolia bark extract standardized for honokiol content, can help to "destress" you without making you sleepy, while a larger dose might have the effect of knocking you out. When compared to pharmaceutical agents such as Valium (diazepam), honokiol appears to be as effective in its antianxiety activity yet not nearly as powerful in its sedative ability. These results have been demonstrated in at least half a dozen animal studies and suggest that magnolia-bark extracts standardized for honokiol content would be an appropriate approach for controlling the detrimental effects of everyday stressors without the tranquilizing side effects of pharmaceutical agents.

No significant toxicity or adverse effects have been associated with traditional use of magnolia bark, but because high doses can cause drowsiness, you might want to hold off on operating that bulldozer or other heavy machinery while you're easing your anxiety with magnolia bark. Typical dosage recommendations range from 250–750 mg per day of an extract standardized for the primary active ingredients (typically 1–2 percent honokiol and magnolol).

KAVA KAVA *(PIPER METHYSTICUM)*

Kava is a root from a pepper plant used for centuries by Pacific islanders (e.g., Fijians, Hawaiians) as a ceremonial intoxicant to help people relax and socialize. More recent uses suggest a role for kava in relieving anxiety and tension. Kava is reported to create a feeling of calmness without dulling the mind or causing alcohol-like hangovers. The active ingredients, chemicals called kavalactones, act as a mild central-nervous-system depressant. The kavalactone content in kava roots can vary significantly from plant to plant (containing between 3 and 20 percent) depending on the growing, harvesting, and processing conditions. Studies of kava, which have largely been conducted in Germany, have found it helpful in alleviating anxiety and other emotional problems related to stress. One study assessed various interpersonal problems and psychological stressors, finding that after four weeks, the group taking kava supplements showed statistically significant decreases in stress in every category measured, in contrast to the placebo group, which showed little variation in any area.

No side effects or withdrawal symptoms have been noted during kava supplementation studies or when people stopped taking the herb. However, a handful of recent case studies from Germany linked kava to liver damage, prompting both the German and Canadian governments to consider removing it from the market. These cases, upon closer examination, turned out to be caused not by kava but rather by combined use of the herb with high levels of alcohol or acetaminophen (Tylenol)—both known to be extremely toxic to the liver.

Because kava depresses the nervous system, it should not be taken with alcohol or in conjunction with antianxiety drugs.

In addition, although kava appears helpful for alleviating cases of mild to moderate anxiety, self-medication with kava is probably not appropriate for individuals with major anxiety conditions. Supplements should provide an extract standardized for kavalactone content, delivering the equivalent of 50–150 mg of kavalactones.

GINSENG

The term "ginseng" refers to a group of adaptogenic herbs from the plant family *Araliacae*. Commonly, "ginseng" refers to "true" ginseng, panax ginseng, which has been used in traditional Chinese medicine for thousands of years as a tonic indicated for its beneficial effects on the central nervous system, protection from stress ulcers, increase of gastrointestinal motility, antifatigue action, enhancement of sexual function, and acceleration of metabolism. Several other "ginsengs" are used as adaptogenic tonics throughout the world; among them are *Panax quinquefolium* (also known as American ginseng), eleutherococcus (also known as Siberian ginseng), and ashwagandha (sometimes called Indian ginseng).

Whether Siberian, panax, or one of the other varieties, the "ginsengs" are generally termed as "adaptogens," defined as therapeutic and restorative tonics generally considered to produce a "balancing" effect on the body. In general, an adaptogen can be thought of as a substance that helps the body to deal with stress.

The active components in panax and American ginseng are thought to be ginsenosides, a family of triterpenoid saponins. In general, most of the top-quality ginseng products, whether whole-root or extract, are standardized for ginsenoside content. The active components in Siberian ginseng are considered to be eleutherosides. It has been theorized that ginseng's action in the body is due to its stimulation of the hypothalamic-pituitary axis to secrete adrenocorticotropic hormone (ACTH). ACTH has the ability to bind directly to brain cells and can affect a variety of behaviors in the body, including motivation, vitality, performance, and arousal.

In a wide range of studies in humans and animals, ginseng improves general indices of stress and mood disturbances, as well as normalizes aspects of metabolism related to controlling cortisol, blood sugar, inflammation, and oxidation.

For the most part, plants in the ginseng family are generally considered quite safe (that's part of the definition they must fulfill to be termed an adaptogen). There are no known drug interactions, contraindications, common allergic reactions, or toxicity to Siberian ginseng, panax ginseng, or American ginseng. A word of caution is recommended, however, for individuals with hypertension, as the stimulatory nature of some ginseng preparations has been reported to increase blood pressure. Additionally, individuals prone to hypoglycemia (low blood sugar) should use ginseng with caution due to the reported effects of ginseng to reduce blood-sugar levels.

Ginseng supplements should be standardized to contain 4–5 percent ginsenosides (for panax ginseng) and 0.5–1.0 percent eleutherosides (for Siberian ginseng). Daily intake of 100–300 mg is recommended to produce adaptogenic and energetic benefits.

PASSIONFLOWER *(PASSIFLORA INCARNATA)*

Passionflower extracts have been studied for their potential ability to decrease anxiety and prolong sleeping time, both of which effects would result in a dramatic reduction in overall cortisol exposure. In very general terms, a number of popular herbs are used to help "take the edge off" after a particularly stressful day. Many of the herbs in this category are found in relaxing herbal teas and include chamomile, melissa, lemon balm, hops, oats, and skullcap. Even though these herbs are widely used to help soothe ragged nerves (again, mostly as herbal teas), none of them have very strong or convincing scientific evidence to support their effectiveness against stress, anxiety, or elevated cortisol levels. That certainly doesn't mean they are useless; after all, a warm cup of tea can sometimes be just the thing to help reduce stress and bring you back to a more relaxed state.

Passionflower may be the exception among the more common herbs found in "relaxation teas," because a number of Indian studies have shown a clear anxiolytic (antianxiety) activity of *Passiflora incarnata* in both animals and humans. Of the few studies in humans, passionflower shows a benefit in treating opiate withdrawal, and a handful of clinical trials have shown passionflower to be as effective as some prescription drugs in the treatment of generalized anxiety. In these studies, the medications tend to have a more rapid onset of action than passionflower (the medications' antianxiety effects "kick in" faster), but the drugs also have more side effects compared to passionflower.

When used as directed, passionflower is quite safe, but high doses can be expected to induce drowsiness and central-nervous-system depression. As such, passionflower should not be combined with barbiturates, antianxiety medications, or antidepressants. The antianxiety effects of passionflower have been confirmed at doses of 400 mg/day, but lower doses of 100–200 mg are generally effective at bedtime for treating insomnia.

RHODIOLA ROSEA

Rhodiola has been used for hundreds of years to treat cold and flulike symptoms, promote longevity, and increase the body's resistance to physical and mental stresses. Like cordyceps and some of the various "ginseng" herbs, rhodiola is typically considered to be an adaptogen and is believed to invigorate the body and mind to increase resistance to a multitude of stresses. The key active constituents in rhodiola are believed to be rosavin, rosarin, rosin, and salidroside.

Studies of rhodiola have shown clear benefits in levels of energy, stamina and endurance, mood, overall mental performance, and resistance to stress.

Rhodiola is considered to be quite safe, with no known contraindications or interactions with other drugs/herbs. General dosage recommendations for rhodiola are typically in the range of 100–300 mg per day.

SCHISANDRA

Schisandra has a long history of use in ancient Chinese medicine as an herb capable of promoting general well-being and enhancing vitality. In addition to its traditional uses for promoting energy and alleviating exhaustion caused by stress, schisandra has historically been taken to strengthen the sex organs, promote mental function, beautify the skin, and treat night sweats, asthma, cough, and insomnia. Schisandra is often touted as a member of the adaptogen family because it contains many chemicals that could support some of the claims made for adaptogens' potentially beneficial effects (including lignans—known to stimulate the immune system, protect the liver, increase the body's ability to cope with stress, and possibly cause a mild sedative effect).

Although schisandra is generally considered to be safe and nontoxic, it may induce uterine muscle contractions at high doses, so pregnant women should not take this herb. Typical dosage recommendations are in the range of 100–500 mg per day.

VALERIAN

Valerian has been used as a medicinal antianxiety herb and sleep aid since the days of the Romans. Although it is unclear which of the numerous compounds is the true "active" ingredient, we know that the whole herb and its extracts (and its combination of compounds) appear to work together in the brain in a manner similar to the action of prescription tranquilizers such as Valium and Halcion. Taken before bedtime, valerian appears to reduce the amount of time it takes to fall asleep—and better/deeper sleep is clearly associated with a reduced cortisol exposure.

Although valerian is considered quite safe, it should be avoided by pregnant and lactating women and should not be consumed by children. Individuals currently taking sedative drugs or antidepressant medications should be advised by their personal physician before taking valerian. Do not take valerian in conjunction with alcohol or other tranquilizers.

Because the activity and strength of valerian preparations can vary significantly from one product to the next, it is recommended to select a standardized product containing 0.5–1.0 percent valerenic acids whenever possible and to follow the directions on the particular product. As a general guideline, approximately 250–500 mg of a 5–6:1 extract can be taken before bed (as a sleep aid) or as needed as a mild tranquilizer.

THEANINE

Theanine is a unique amino acid found in the leaves of green tea (*Camellia sinensis*). Theanine is quite different from the polyphenol and catechin antioxidants for which green tea is typically consumed. In fact, through the natural production of polyphenols, the tea plant converts theanine into catechins. This means that tea leaves harvested during one part of the growing season may be high in catechins (good for antioxidant benefits), while leaves harvested during another time of year may be higher in theanine (good for antistress and cortisol-controlling effects). Three to four cups of green tea are expected to contain 100–200 mg of theanine.

The unique aspect of theanine is that it acts as a nonsedating relaxant to help increase the brain's production of alpha waves (those associated with "relaxed alertness"). This makes theanine extremely effective for combating tension, stress, and anxiety—without inducing drowsiness. By increasing the brain's output of alpha waves, theanine is thought to control anxiety, increase mental focus, improve concentration, and promote creativity. Research studies are quite clear on the facts that people who produce more alpha brain waves also have less anxiety, that highly creative people generate more alpha waves when faced with a problem to solve, and that elite athletes tend to produce a burst of alpha waves on the left side of their brains during their best performances.

No adverse side effects are associated with theanine consumption, making it one of the leading natural choices for promoting relaxation without the sedating effects of depressant drugs. Clinical studies show that theanine is effective in dosages ranging from 50 to 200 mg per day—about what you would find in two to four cups of green tea. Because theanine reaches its maximum levels in the blood between thirty minutes and two hours after taking it, it can be used both as a daily antistress and mental-focus regimen and "as needed" as a supplement during stressful times.

. . . .
.
.

CHAPTER 7

Supplements for the Control of Oxidation

Antioxidants are important for controlling the activity of the highly reactive oxygen molecules known as free radicals, because unchecked free-radical activity is what leads to the cellular damage known as oxidation and the cycle of glycation and inflammation that follows, causing additional damage and dysfunction. When it comes to antioxidant supplementation, however, it is the overall collection of several antioxidants that is important, rather than any single "super" antioxidant. This is what scientists call the "antioxidant network," and it is made up of five major classes of antioxidants: vitamin E, vitamin C, carotenoids, bioflavonoids, and thiols. Your cells need representatives from each of these categories in order to mount the strongest antioxidant defense.

Think of it this way: If you had the best home run hitter in the world, but poor pitching and fielding, then your baseball team would not be the best. The same thing applies to your antioxidant defenses. Green tea, vitamin E, pine bark, and beta-carotene are all wonderful antioxidants on their own, but combining them to create a network that works together in different parts of the body and against different types of free radicals is the most effective way to go. Some of the top picks are beta-carotene (natural), lycopene, lutein, vitamin E (natural), vitamin C, alpha-lipoic acid, green tea, selenium, zinc, grape seed, and pine bark. But there are many other choices of nutrients and herbal extracts and plant extracts that also possess wonderful antioxidant properties, several of which are summarized in this chapter.

ANTIOXIDANTS
A GENERAL DISCUSSION

The term "antioxidant" refers to the ability possessed by numerous vitamins, minerals, and other phytochemicals to serve as protection against the damaging effects of highly reactive molecules known as free radicals. Free radicals have the ability to chemically react with, and damage, many structures in the body. Particularly susceptible to oxidative damage are the cell membranes of virtually all cells, especially those in the skin, because of the skin's high lipid content and its vulnerability to ultraviolet rays from the sun.

The free-radical theory of aging and disease promotion holds that through a gradual accumulation of microscopic damage to our cell membranes, DNA, tissue structures, and enzyme systems, we begin to lose function and become predisposed to disease. In the case of athletes and other avid exercisers, oxidative damage may be elevated due to increased production of free radicals during intense activity. Although the body increases its production of endogenous antioxidant enzymes (glutathione peroxidase, catalase, superoxide dismutase) when it is under stress, it can be theorized that supplemental levels of exogenous or dietary antioxidants may be warranted to prevent excessive oxidative damage to muscles, mitochondria, and other structures.

Thousands of studies have clearly documented the beneficial effects of dozens of antioxidant nutrients. There is certainly no shortage of nutrients and phytochemicals that possess significant antioxidant activity in the test tube. Increased dietary intake of these nutrients—for example, vitamins C and E, minerals such as selenium, and various phytonutrients such as extracts from grape seed, pine bark, and green tea—have all been linked to reduced rates of oxidative damage, as well as to reduced incidence of chronic illnesses such as heart disease and cancer.

At the typically recommended levels, the majority of antioxidants appear to be quite safe. For example, vitamin E, one of the most powerful membrane-bound antioxidants, also has one of the best safety profiles. Doses of 100–400 IU (international units) have been linked to significant cardiovascular benefits with no side effects. Vitamin C, another powerful antioxidant, can help to protect and restore the antioxidant activity of vitamin E, and it is considered safe up to doses of 500–1,000 mg. Higher doses of vitamin C are not recommended because of concerns that such levels may cause an "unbalancing" of the oxidative systems and actually promote oxidative damage instead of preventing it. Another popular antioxidant, beta-carotene, is somewhat controversial as a dietary supplement. Although diets high in fruits and vegetables might deliver approximately 5–6 mg of carotenes daily, these would include a mixture of beta-carotene and other naturally occurring carotenoids. Concern was raised several years ago by studies in which high-dose beta-carotene supplements appeared to promote lung cancer in heavy smokers. Those studies provided unbalanced synthetic beta-carotene supplements of 20–60 mg—about five to ten times the levels that could reasonably be expected in the diet.

The four key nutritional antioxidants—vitamins C and E, beta-carotene, and selenium—are well studied, widely available as dietary supplements, and relatively inexpensive. As mentioned above, there are a multitude of fruit and vegetable phytonutrient extracts available that also possess significant antioxidant activity.

VITAMIN A

Vitamin A is a fat-soluble vitamin that is part of a family of compounds including retinol, retinal, and beta-carotene. Beta-carotene (discussed in more detail below) is also known as "pro-vitamin A," because it can be converted into vitamin A when additional levels are required. Vitamin A is found only in animal products; food sources include organ meats such as liver and kidney, egg yolks, butter, fortified dairy products (e.g., milk and some margarines), and cod liver oil.

Vitamin A is needed by all of the body's tissues for general growth and repair processes; it is especially important for bone formation, healthy skin and hair, night vision, and the proper functioning of the immune system. Vitamin A may help boost immune-system function and resistance to infection. Vitamin A derivatives are widely used in cosmetics and dermatological treatments for skin preparations designed to combat skin aging and treat acne.

Be aware that as a fat-soluble vitamin, vitamin A can be stored in the body and levels can build up over time. Possible toxicity can result with high-dose supplementation (50,000 IU/day), leading to vomiting, headaches, joint pain, skin irritation, gastrointestinal distress, and hair loss.

Extreme caution should be exercised during pregnancy, as high-dose vitamin A has been associated with teratogenic effects (birth defects) on the fetuses of pregnant women. A maximum daily intake of 5,000 IU of vitamin A is suggested during pregnancy.

The FDA's recommended daily value (DV) for vitamin A is 5,000 IU for adults. Children should consume no more than 3,500 IU daily. Although there is no established DV for beta-carotene, a daily intake of 5–20 mg has been advocated by some nutrition experts.

SPIRULINA

The term "spirulina" includes various species of primitive, unicellular blue-green algae. These microscopic plants grow naturally in lakes rich in salt, particularly in Central and South America and in Africa. The bulk of these microscopic aquatic plants used in supplements are grown and harvested in outdoor tanks in California, Hawaii, Australia, and Asia.

Because spirulina is a whole organism, it contains many important nutrients, including vitamins, minerals, essential fatty acids, and all of the essential amino acids (those which the human body cannot produce). It also contains chlorophyll and carotenoids, both of which have been receiving quite a bit of attention for their antioxidant properties. Because spirulina contains high levels of protein and low levels of fat, powder made from this alga is often mixed with juice as a supplement to low-calorie diets. Spirulina is also a rich source of gamma linoleic acid (GLA), an essential acid found in everyday foods, as well as in herbal extracts such as evening primrose oil (good for its anti-inflammatory effects).

Studies in animals fed large quantities of spirulina have shown that it is not toxic, and that it causes virtually no adverse health effects. Dosage recommendations for spirulina are in the range of 2–3 grams daily.

VITAMIN C (ASCORBIC ACID)

Vitamin C, also known as ascorbic acid, is a water-soluble vitamin needed by the body for hundreds of vital metabolic reactions. Good food sources of vitamin C include all citrus fruits (oranges, grapefruit, lemons), as well as many other fruits and vegetables, including strawberries, tomatoes, broccoli, Brussels sprouts, peppers, and cantaloupe.

Perhaps the best-known function of vitamin C is as one of the key nutritional antioxidants. As a water-soluble vitamin, ascorbic acid performs its antioxidant functions within the aqueous compartments of the blood and inside cells and can help restore the antioxidant potential of vitamin E (a fat-soluble antioxidant).

Vitamin C also functions as an essential cofactor for the enzymes involved in the synthesis of collagen, the chief structural protein in connective tissues such as bones, cartilage, and skin. As such, vitamin C is often recommended for wound healing and as an added ingredient in supplements designed for promoting healthy skin.

As a preventive against infections such as influenza and other viruses, vitamin C is thought to strengthen the cell membranes, thereby preventing entrance of the virus into the interior of the cell. Support of immune-cell function—an effect that may help fight infections in their early stages—is also a key role performed by vitamin C. The combined effects of cellular strengthening, collagen synthesis, and antioxidant protection are thought to account for the multifaceted approach through which vitamin C helps to maintain health.

In most cases, it appears that while the most important and dramatic preventive effects of vitamin C supplementation will be experienced by individuals with low vitamin C intakes, those with an average daily consumption from foods may also benefit from supplemental levels. In support of an elevated vitamin C intake, an expert scientific panel recently recommended increasing vitamin C intake to protect cells from oxidation.

As a water-soluble vitamin, ascorbic acid is extremely safe even at relatively high doses (because most of the excess is excreted in the urine). At high doses (over 1,000 mg/day), some people can experience gastrointestinal side effects such as stomach cramps, nausea, and diarrhea and may have an increased risk of developing kidney stones.

Although the suggested daily intake (DRI, or Dietary Reference Intake) for vitamin C has recently been raised from 60 mg to 75–90 mg (higher for pregnant and lactating women), it is well established that almost everybody can benefit from even higher levels. For example, the vitamin C recommendation for cigarette smokers is 100–200 mg per day because smoking destroys vitamin C in the body. Although vitamin C is well absorbed, the percent absorbed from supplements decreases with higher dosages; optimal absorption is achieved by taking several small doses (about 200 mg per dose) throughout the day, for a total daily intake of 200–1,000 mg. Full blood and tissue saturation is achieved with daily intakes of 200–500 mg per day, divided among two or three doses.

VITAMIN E (TOCOPHEROLS AND TOCOTRIENOLS)

Vitamin E is actually a family of related compounds known as tocopherols and tocotrienols. Although alpha-tocopherol is the most common form found in dietary supplements, vitamin E also exists with slightly different chemical structures as beta-, gamma-, and delta-tocopherol and as alpha-, beta-, gamma-, and delta-tocotrienol. Natural forms of all eight structures are important for overall health.

Vitamin E can be obtained as a supplement in natural or synthetic form. In most cases, the natural and synthetic forms of vitamins and minerals are identical, but in the case of vitamin E, the natural form is clearly superior in terms of absorption and retention in the body. The natural form of alpha-tocopherol is known as "d-alpha-tocopherol," whereas the synthetic form is called "dl-alpha-tocopherol." The synthetic "dl-" form is the most common form found in dietary supplements, although many manufacturers are switching over to the more potent (and more expensive) natural "d-" form.

Dietary sources of vitamin E include vegetable oils, margarine, nuts, seeds, avocados, and wheat germ. Safflower oil contains a good amount of vitamin E (about two-thirds of the DRI in a quarter cup), but there is very little vitamin E in either corn oil or soybean oil. For individuals watching their dietary fat consumption, vitamin E intake is likely to be low, due to a reduced intake of foods with high fat content. You'd need to eat about sixty almonds to get the DRI for vitamin E and several hundred almonds to get the amount of the vitamin associated with health benefits (200–400 IU).

Of the different types of vitamin E, the alpha-tocopherol form is typically considered the "gold standard" in terms of antioxidant activity—although the most recent research suggests that the other chemical forms may possess equivalent or superior antioxidant protection. Several studies published over the last few years have clearly shown that natural vitamin E, the "d-" form, is about two to three times more bioavailable than the synthetic "dl-" vitamin E. The natural form of the vitamin is extracted from vegetable oils, mostly from soybeans, which are cheap and plentiful in the United States. Synthetic vitamin E, by contrast, is manufactured from chemicals related to petroleum products, which results in a blend in which only one-eighth of the mixture is the powerful "d-" isomer.

A wide variety of epidemiological and prospective studies have shown health benefits associated with higher than average vitamin E consumption. In most cases, the levels of vitamin E intake required for heart, lung, eye, and cancer protection are ten to thirty times higher than the current DRI levels. Although high-dose alpha-tocopherol supplements are clearly a powerful antioxidant measure, concern has recently been raised because such supplements may displace body stores of the other, naturally occurring, vitamin E forms.

Overall, the majority of evidence indicates that a balanced intake of each of the naturally occurring forms of vitamin E may be the most prudent approach in terms of overall health benefits. For example, high-dose "alpha-form" supplements can reduce body stores of gamma-tocopherol, whereas a fifty-fifty intake of each maintains elevated tissue stores of both. Such findings are potentially important, given that gamma-tocopherol is the major form of vitamin E in the American diet and has been found, in a test-tube study, to inhibit lipid peroxidation (cell membrane damage) more effectively than alpha-tocopherol. This could mean that the different vitamin E forms may complement each other in the body.

Side effects associated with vitamin E supplements are exceedingly rare. Unlike other fat-soluble vitamins (A, D, and K), vitamin E is relatively nontoxic, even at doses of many times the current recommended levels. A caution is advised, however, for individuals at risk for prolonged bleeding, such as those taking anticoagulant medications, because vitamin E supplements can decrease blood-clotting ability (via reduced platelet aggregation) and prolong bleeding time.

The daily value (DV) for vitamin E is 30 IU, but most research studies show that optimal intakes associated with health benefits are in the range of 100–400 IU, an amount that is unrealistic to obtain from foods.

BETA-CAROTENE

Beta-carotene is part of a large family of compounds known as carotenoids. The carotenoid group includes over six hundred members, including the antioxidants lycopene and lutein. Carotenoids are widely distributed in fruits and vegetables and are responsible, along with flavonoids, for contributing the color to many plants. (As discussed earlier in the book, remember that a nutritional rule of thumb is "the brighter the better.") In terms of nutrition, beta-carotene's primary role is as a precursor to vitamin A: The body can convert beta-carotene into vitamin A as needed. It is important to note that beta-carotene and vitamin A are often described in the same breath —almost as if they were the same compound, which they are not. Although beta-carotene can be converted into vitamin A in the body, there are important differences in terms of action and safety between the two compounds. Beta-carotene, like most carotenoids, is a powerful antioxidant and is especially effective at preventing sunlight damage to skin. The best food sources for beta-carotene are brightly colored fruits and veggies, such as cantaloupe, apricots, carrots, red peppers, sweet potatoes, winter squash, and dark leafy greens.

It is important to note that the vast majority of the scientific evidence for the health benefits of beta-carotene comes from studies that looked at *food* sources of beta-carotene (and other carotenoids, often referred to as "mixed" carotenoids)—not supplements. From population (epidemiological) studies, we know that a high consumption of fruits and vegetables is associated with a significant reduction in many diseases—especially several forms of cancer (lung, stomach, colon, breast, prostate, and bladder). Because the data suggest that the "active" components in a plant-based diet may be carotenoids, and because beta-carotene is the chief carotenoid in our diets, it was widely believed until about the mid-1990s that the majority of the health benefits attributable to fruits and vegetables may be due to beta-carotene.

One of the largest epidemiological studies, the Physicians' Health Study (PHS, which involved over twenty-two thousand male physicians), found that while high levels of carotenoids obtained from the diet were associated with reduced cancer risk, beta-carotene from supplements (about 25 mg/day) had no effect on cancer risk. A possible explanation for this finding may be that while purified beta-carotene may contribute some antioxidant benefits, a "blend" of carotenoids (and/or other compounds in fruits and veggies) is probably even more important for preventing cancer. It may even be possible that isolated beta-carotene supplements could interfere with absorption or metabolism of other beneficial carotenoids from the diet.

Unfortunately, intervention studies that have looked at purified synthetic beta-carotene supplements (not mixed carotenoids) have not cleared up any of the confusion. In

1994, the results from a supplementation study of almost thirty thousand subjects (ATBC, the Alpha-Tocopherol and Beta-Carotene study) showed not only that beta-carotene supplementation (20 mg/day for five to eight years) did *not* prevent lung cancer in high-risk subjects (longtime male smokers), but that it actually caused an increase in lung cancer risk by almost 20 percent. This same study also found a 10 percent increase in heart disease and a 20 percent increase in strokes among the beta-carotene users. In 1996, another large study (CARET, the Beta-Carotene and Retinol Efficacy Trial) found virtually the same thing; subjects who received beta-carotene showed almost 50 percent more cases of lung cancer. These results were so alarming that the National Cancer Institute decided to halt the forty-million-dollar study nearly two years early. The ATBC study examined longtime heavy smokers, while the CARET study looked at present and former smokers, as well as workers exposed to asbestos—all of which can be considered "high-risk" populations for developing lung cancer (which may or may not have contributed to the surprising study results).

On the positive side, beta-carotene has been successfully used for more than fifteen years to treat inherited photosensitivity diseases, such as erythropoietic protoporphyria (EPP), and other skin conditions. For this reason beta-carotene has found its way into a variety of topical and internally consumed products meant for skin protection. In Europe, one of the most popular uses for carotenoid supplements (primarily lycopene and beta-carotene) is as "inside-out" skin protection during the summer sunbathing months.

At recommended dosages, beta-carotene is thought to be quite safe—although, as mentioned, at least two large studies have shown that high-dose beta-carotene (20–50 mg per day) can increase the risk of heart disease and cancer in smokers. Other reported side effects from high-dose beta-carotene sup-

plements (100,000 IU or 60 mg per day) include nausea, diarrhea, and a yellow-orange tinge to the skin, especially in the
hands and feet, which fades at lower doses. The safest way to
get your beta-carotene and other carotenoids is from eating a
wide variety of fruits and vegetables.

If you choose to take beta-carotene in supplement form,
the supplements are relatively inexpensive and widely available. They contain both synthetic and natural sources of beta-
carotene. The natural forms typically come from algae (*Duna-
liella salina*), fungi (*Blakeslea trispora*), or palm oil. In terms of
conversion to vitamin A, the "trans-" form of beta-carotene
has the maximum conversion rate. Nearly all synthetic beta-
carotene comes in the "trans-" form (98 percent), while natural sources vary in the form of beta-carotene they provide.
(The different forms are known as isomers.) Among natural
forms of beta-carotene, the fungal form provides the highest
concentration of trans beta-carotene (94 percent), followed
by algae sources (64 percent) and palm oil sources (34 percent)—so from the perspective of vitamin A conversion, either the synthetic form or the fungal form of beta-carotene
will provide the highest conversion into active vitamin A.
From a "mixed" carotenoid perspective, however, beta-carotene derived from algae also provides the "cis-" isomer of beta-
carotene (about 31 percent), as well as alpha-carotene (3–4
percent) and other carotenoids (1–2 percent). Beta-carotene
derived form palm oil provides the most balanced mixture of
carotenoid isomers (34 percent trans-beta, 27 percent cis-beta,
30 percent alpha, and 9 percent other carotenoids)—but it
also has the lowest vitamin A conversion, because it only provides 34 percent as the trans form.

Three milligrams of beta-carotene supplies 5,000 IU of vitamin A. Although beta-carotene supplements are commonly
available in doses of 25,000 IU (15 mg) per day, and many
people consume as much as 100,000 IU (60 mg) per day, the

current state of the scientific literature does not support doses of beta-carotene much higher than those levels recommended for supplying vitamin A precursors (about 5,000–10,000 IU per day of beta-carotene, or 3–6 mg).

GREEN TEA *(CAMELLIA SINENSIS)*

Green tea is the second-most consumed beverage in the world (water is the first) and has been used medicinally for centuries in India and China. Green tea is prepared by picking the leaves, lightly steaming them, and allowing them to dry. Black tea, the most popular type of tea in the United States, is made by allowing the leaves to ferment before drying. Due to differences in the fermentation process, a portion of the plant's active compounds is destroyed in black tea, but these compounds remain active in green tea. The active constituents in green tea are a family of polyphenols (catechins) and flavonols that possess potent antioxidant activity. Tannins, large polyphenol molecules, form the bulk of the active compounds in green tea, with catechins comprising nearly 90 percent. Several catechins are present in significant quantities: epicatechin (EC), epigallocatechin (EGC), epicatechin gallate (ECG), and epigallocatechin gallate (EGCG). EGCG makes up about 10–50 percent of the total catechin content and appears to be the most powerful of the catechins; its antioxidant activity is about twenty-five to one hundred times more potent than that of vitamins C and E. A cup of green tea may provide 10–40 mg of polyphenols and has antioxidant activity greater than a serving of broccoli, spinach, carrots, or strawberries. A number of commercial green tea extracts are standardized to total polyphenol content and/or EGCG content.

From laboratory findings, it is clear that green tea is an effective antioxidant, that it provides protection from experimentally induced DNA damage, and that it may slow or halt the initiation and progression of cancerous tumor growth.

Several epidemiological studies show an association between consumption of total flavonoids in the diet and reduced risk for cancer and heart disease. Men with the highest consumption of flavonoids from fruits and vegetables have approximately half the risk of heart disease and cancer, compared to those with the lowest intake. The primary catechin in green tea, EGCG, appears to inhibit the growth of cancer cells and play a role in stimulating apoptosis (programmed cell death), both of which are crucial aspects of cancer prevention.

Consumption of as much as twenty cups per day of green tea has not been associated with any significant side effects. In high doses, teas that contain caffeine may lead to restlessness, insomnia, and tachycardia. Decaffeinated versions of green tea and green tea extracts are available, but due to differences in caffeine extraction methods, the amounts of phenolic/catechin compounds can vary between extracts. Be sure to choose an extract that is decaffeinated as well as standardized for total polyphenol content and/or catechin concentrations. In addition, individuals taking aspirin or other anticoagulant medications (including vitamin E and ginkgo biloba) on a daily basis should be aware of the possible inhibition of platelet aggregation (blood clotting) associated with green tea. In some cases, green tea may prolong bleeding times.

Typical dosage recommendations are for 125–500 mg/day —preferably of an extract standardized to at least 40 percent polyphenols (roughly equivalent to four to ten cups of brewed green tea).

FLAVONOIDS/POLYPHENOLS

Polyphenols are a class of phytochemicals found in high concentrations in wine, tea, grapes, and a wide variety of other plants. They have been associated with prevention of heart disease and cancer. Phenolic compounds are responsible for the brightly colored pigments of many fruits and vegetables;

these pigments protect plants from diseases and ultraviolet light and help prevent damage to seeds until they germinate. One of the more nutritionally important classes of polyphenols, the flavonoids, is widely distributed in plant foods. This class includes the following phytochemicals:

- Lignans (nuts, whole-grain cereals)
- Proanthocyanins (grapes, pine bark)
- Anthocyanins/anthocyanidins (brightly colored fruits and vegetables, berries)
- Isoflavones: genistein/daidzein (soybeans)
- Catechins (tea, grapes, wine)
- Tannins (tea, nuts)
- Quercetin (grapes, wine, onions)
- Naringenin/hesperidin (citrus fruits)

Polyphenols, particularly the flavonoids, are among the most potent plant antioxidants. They can form complexes with reactive metals such as iron, zinc, and copper, reducing their absorption by the body. At first glance, a reduction in nutrient absorption may seem to be a negative side effect, but excess levels of these elements (metal cations) in the body can promote the generation of free radicals and contribute to the oxidative damage of cell membranes and cellular DNA. In addition to their chelating effect on metal cations, polyphenols also function as potent free-radical scavengers within the body, where they neutralize free radicals before they can cause cellular damage.

Epidemiologic studies have shown a relationship between high dietary intakes of phenolics and reduced risk of cardiovascular disease and cancer. You've undoubtedly heard of the "French paradox," by which regular, moderate consumption of red wine, which is rich in polyphenols, is associated with low rates of coronary artery disease, an oxidative and inflammatory condition. In general, polyphenols (flavonoids) are thought to deliver health benefits by several mechanisms, including: (1) direct free-radical quenching, (2) protection and regeneration of other dietary antioxidants (e.g., vitamin E), (3) chelation of metal ions, and (4) a generalized anti-inflammatory effect.

No significant side effects are evident from regular consumption of polyphenol- or flavonoid-containing dietary supplements. Fruits and vegetables can vary significantly in total polyphenol content, depending on the part of the plant used, cultivation and harvesting methods, degree of ripeness, storage conditions, and processing methods. Following dietary recommendations for five or more servings of fruits and vegetables daily would result in a total flavonoid intake of about 150–300 mg per day. Supplemental intake should be in this range; specific recommendations will vary depending on the compound in question (e.g., grape seed, pine bark, green tea, etc.).

LYCOPENE

Lycopene is a carotenoid (like beta-carotene) that is responsible for giving tomatoes their red color. Although there are about six hundred carotenoids, lycopene is the most abundant form found in the U.S. diet (beta-carotene is number two). More than 80 percent of the lycopene consumed in the United States comes from tomato sauce, pizza, and ketchup. The lycopene content of tomatoes can be influenced dramatically during the ripening process, and large differences are noted between various types of tomatoes (e.g., red varieties have more lycopene than yellow ones). The bioavailability of lycopene is increased following cooking, so processed tomato products such as ketchup, tomato juice, and pizza sauce have more bioavailable lycopene than do fresh tomatoes.

Because lycopene is a potent antioxidant and seems to inhibit the growth of cancer cells, it is logical that a higher intake of this carotenoid may indeed be associated with reduced incidence of cancer. Likewise, lycopene is known to play a role, along with beta-carotene, in protecting the skin from the damaging effects of ultraviolet radiation.

The theory behind lycopene's cancer-preventive benefits is logical. Indeed, several epidemiologic studies have shown that consumption of foods high in lycopene is associated with lower rates of prostate cancer. Furthermore, plasma lycopene levels are reduced by about 40–50 percent in smokers, whose lungs are exposed to a high degree of oxidative damage. Dietary supplements containing 20–40 mg of lycopene have been shown to reduce DNA damage in white blood cells—probably due to the reduction in oxidative damage to DNA and lipoproteins. As an antioxidant, lycopene is twice as effective as beta-carotene in protecting white blood cells from membrane damage caused by free radicals.

No significant adverse side effects are associated with regular consumption of supplemental levels of lycopene, but owing to the controversy surrounding high doses of supplemental beta-carotene (which appears to increase lung cancer risk; see above), doses of lycopene should remain in the range of levels attainable from a diet high in tomato-based products (20–40 mg/day).

LUTEIN/ZEAXANTHIN

Lutein and zeaxanthin are carotenoids found in highest concentration in the macular region of the eye (the back of the eyeball where the retina is located), where they are believed to help filter out damaging blue light and prevent free-radical damage to the delicate structures located there. These carotenoids also are known to concentrate in the skin, where they can protect collagen and elastin from the same UV radiation that bombards the eye. Anybody who spends time outdoors exposed to the sun should be concerned with the potential for ultraviolet radiation to damage the delicate structures in the eyes and the skin, but antioxidants can provide some protection against this source of oxidative destruction.

Lutein and zeaxanthin are yellow pigments found in high concentrations in egg yolks, yellow fruits and vegetables, and dark-green leafy vegetables. In particular, spinach, kale, and collard greens contain high levels of these two carotenoids— so high that individuals who consume large amounts of spinach reduce their risk of developing age-related macular degeneration (ARMD) by almost 90 percent.

Both lutein and zeaxanthin seem to reduce oxidative damage and protect tissues via a two-step process. First, both of these carotenoids are absorbed from the diet into the bloodstream and eventually end up concentrated specifically in the eye and the skin. Next, as mentioned, the high levels of these carotenoids in these tissues serve to protect the tissues by minimizing free-radical damage and by absorbing harmful blue-light rays.

Most studies on lutein and zeaxanthin have been conducted in patients with eye problems, but the same mechanisms are at work in your skin. Several observational studies have shown that high dietary intakes of lutein and zeaxanthin (from spinach, broccoli, and eggs) are associated with a significant reduction in the risk for cataract (up to 20 percent) and for ARMD (up to 40 percent). One study has shown that dietary supplementation with lutein (30 mg/day for 140 days) elevates serum lutein levels by ten times, increases macular pigment density by 20–40 percent, and reduces transmission of blue light to the eye's photoreceptors by 30–40 percent. Another study showed that daily egg yolk consumption can increase plasma levels of lutein by 28–50 percent and levels of zeaxanthin by 114–142 percent. A multicenter clinical study (the Eye Disease Case-Control Study) compared 356 patients with advanced ARMD, ages fifty-five to eighty, to 520 control subjects. The researchers found that the risk for ARMD was reduced by over 40 percent with a high dietary intake of carotenoids. In particular, both lutein and zeaxanthin were strongly associated with a reduced risk for the development of macular degeneration.

There are no known adverse side effects associated with dietary supplements containing lutein or zeaxanthin, when used at recommended levels. Most supplements should be taken with a meal in order to lessen the chance of causing stomach upset and to increase their digestion and absorption (bioavailability).

Diets providing about 6 mg of lutein per day can reduce oxidative damage to the eye and ARMD prevalence by nearly half. Eating more of the carotenoid-rich foods mentioned above should be your first step to increase lutein intake. Unfortunately, recent diet surveys have indicated that consumption of these foods is insufficient in the two groups at highest risk for ARMD: women and the elderly. Since many carotenoids are cleared from the body rapidly, you may want to consider splitting your daily intake of lutein and zeaxanthin into two doses: 3 mg with breakfast and 3 mg with dinner.

GOTU KOLA *(CENTELLA ASIATICA)*

In India and Indonesia, gotu kola has a long history of use to promote wound healing and treat skin diseases. In Europe, extracts are prescribed by doctors for the treatment of wound-healing defects. Gotu kola should not be confused with kola nut, which is completely unrelated and is often used in dietary supplements as a "natural" source of caffeine.

Gotu kola contains a blend of compounds, including at least three triterpenes (asiatic acid, madecassic acid, and asiaticoside) that appear to have antioxidant benefits and an ability to stimulate collagen synthesis for tissue regeneration.

Perhaps the best indication for gotu kola is its ability to improve symptoms of varicose veins (which are caused by a defect in collagen turnover), and particularly those of overall discomfort, tiredness, and swelling. In human studies, gotu kola extract (30–180 mg/day for four weeks) leads to improvements in a number of measurements of vein function (foot swelling, ankle edema, and fluid leakage from the veins—all of which indicate a more robust cycle of collagen synthesis and repair) compared to placebo.

Gotu kola appears to have a generally beneficial effect on connective tissues, where it may improve the structure and function of the tissue in the body, keeping veins stronger and also possibly reducing the symptoms of other connective-tissue diseases. In one animal study, asiatic acid and asiaticoside were the most active of the three triterpenes—but all three were effective in stimulating collagen synthesis and glycosaminoglycan synthesis. Radiation injury to the skin of rats can be reduced by treatment with madecassol, one of the triterpene compounds in gotu kola, suggesting skin regeneration and anti-inflammatory activity.

The activity of asiaticoside has been studied in normal, as well as in delayed-type wound healing. In one animal study (guinea pig punch wounds), topical applications of asiaticoside (0.2 percent solution) produced a 56 percent increase in hydroxyproline and a 57 percent increase in tensile strength, increased collagen content, and better epithelization. In diabetic rats, in whom healing is delayed, topical application of 0.4 percent solution of asiaticoside over punch wounds increased hydroxyproline content, tensile strength, collagen content, and epithelization, thereby facilitating healing. In each of these studies, asiaticoside was also shown to be active by the oral route (at a dose of 1 mg/kg of body weight), suggesting that gotu kola may work by stimulating synthesis of collagen and increasing connective-tissue strength.

Other studies have indicated that asiaticoside has an antioxidant effect. When applied topically (0.2 percent solution) twice daily for seven days to skin wounds in rats, results show an increase in both enzymatic and nonenzymatic antioxidants in newly formed tissues, namely, superoxide dismutase (35 percent), catalase (67 percent), glutathione peroxidase (49 percent), vitamin E (77 percent), and ascorbic acid (36 percent). It also results in a several-fold decrease in lipid peroxide levels (69 percent) as measured in terms of thiobarbituric acid reactive substance (TBARS). This enhancement of antioxidant levels at an initial stage of healing may be an important contributory factor in the healing properties of gotu kola.

When taken orally, gotu kola appears to be nontoxic, and it seldom causes any side effects, though there is some anecdotal evidence that the herb may result in elevated bloodsugar levels, an effect that could be of concern to individuals with diabetes.

Typical dosage recommendations for gotu kola are in the range of 60–180 mg/day, usually consumed in divided doses (20–60 mg three times daily for at least four weeks). It is important to look for an extract standardized to contain triterpene compounds—typically 30–40 percent and including asiaticoside, asiatic acid, madecassic acid, and madecassoside. These compounds usually occur at only 1–4 percent in the whole herb.

. . . .
. :
:

CHAPTER 8

Supplements for the Control of AGEs

When most people think of controlling blood sugar, they automatically think of diabetes, a chronic disease that affects about twenty million Americans. There are at least double that number—more than forty million Americans—who have what might be called "prediabetes," a dysfunctional or suboptimal control of blood sugar. Most of these people are completely unaware that their blood-sugar levels are fluctuating wildly throughout the day, but they clearly feel the effects in terms of fatigue, problems concentrating, constant hunger, weight gain—and, yes, accelerated skin aging (mostly via glycation, but also via oxidation and inflammation).

Control of blood sugar—and the excessive glycation that can result from improper control—can benefit greatly from a number of the dietary supplements outlined below.

CHROMIUM

Chromium is a trace mineral that is essential for normal insulin function. (Insulin is the hormone that causes blood sugar, or glucose, to be absorbed into cells for metabolization by the body.) Dietary studies indicate that most people in the United States and other industrialized countries don't get enough chromium, and deficiencies appear to be even more common in people with diabetes and problems with blood-sugar control. Chromium is an essential trace mineral that aids in glucose metabolism, regulation of insulin levels, and maintenance of healthy blood levels of cholesterol and other lipids. Chromium forms part of a compound in the body known as glucose tolerance factor (GTF), which is involved in regulating the actions of insulin in maintaining blood-sugar levels and possibly in helping to control appetite. Food sources for chromium include brewer's yeast, whole-grain cereals, broccoli, prunes, mushrooms, and beer.

Chromium deficiency is known to lead to glucose intolerance and insulin resistance, symptoms commonly encountered in people with diabetes. Since chromium helps regulate the actions of insulin (as a constituent of glucose tolerance factor), chromium supplements may help support the many functions of insulin in the body, such as maintaining blood-sugar levels.

Many clinical studies support the benefits and safety of chromium supplementation for normalizing blood sugar. Supplemental chromium can lower blood insulin levels, improve glucose tolerance, and decrease systemic levels of glycation. Experts from the U.S. Department of Agriculture at the Beltsville Human Nutrition Research Center in Maryland recommend chromium supplementation in daily amounts of 200–1,000 mcg (micrograms) for optimal blood-sugar control. Clinical studies show that the inorganic forms of chromium, such as chromium chloride, are not as effective as the organic or chelated forms, such as chromium polynicotinate, picolinate, glycine-niacin chelate, GTF chromium, and chromium yeast.

VANADIUM

Vanadium is another trace element involved in promoting normal insulin function. A normal diet typically provides about 10–30 mcg of vanadium per day. Although there is currently no DRI established, this amount appears to be adequate for most healthy adults. Supplemental forms of vanadium are usually vanadyl or vanadate forms. Vanadium is thought to play a role in metabolism of carbohydrates and may have functions in cholesterol and blood lipid metabolism. In diabetics, vanadium supplements may have a positive effect in regulating glucose levels. Food sources of vanadium include seafood, mushrooms, some cereals, and soybeans.

Vanadium or its most common supplemental form, vanadyl sulfate, is thought to mimic the physiological effects of insulin through a mechanism that remains unclear. Through this insulin-mimetic effect, vanadium is thought to promote glycogen synthesis and maintain glucose levels. Vanadyl sulfate supplements have been shown to normalize glucose levels and reduce glycosylated hemoglobin levels and can reduce fasting glucose levels by about 20 percent.

Limited information is available about vanadium's toxicity. Traditionally, vanadium is considered quite safe in humans because of its poor absorption. In one safety study, 100 mg of vanadyl sulfate (a *huge* dose) was given to diabetic subjects for four weeks (50 mg twice per day). Gastrointestinal side effects were experienced by 75 percent of the subjects. It is thought that prolonged exposure to excessive vanadium could cause muscle cramps, emotional depression, and damage to the nervous system and other organs. There is no daily value (DV) or dietary reference intake (DRI) for vanadium, although it is now considered an essential trace mineral. Supplements of approximately 10–30 mcg per day are thought to satisfy the body's needs.

ZINC

Zinc is an essential trace mineral for immune function, antioxidant protection, and reproduction. Three out of four of us do not meet the recommended intakes for zinc. Zinc supplementation is especially important for reducing glycation because it also promotes normal insulin function. However, to avoid unwanted nutrient interactions, zinc should not be supplemented in high doses (above 45 mg daily) and is best taken in balance with other trace elements, such as copper (2 mg of copper for every 15 mg of zinc).

ALPHA-LIPOIC ACID

Alpha-lipoic acid has been established by many European and U.S. studies as an important antioxidant *and* blood-sugar controller. It has been called the "universal" antioxidant, because it reacts with many different free radicals. Alpha-lipoic acid supplementation enhances insulin action and can reduce or reverse oxidative nerve damage from elevated blood-sugar levels. In conjunction with other antioxidants, such as vitamin E, alpha-lipoic acid may be doubly helpful in patients with diabetes. By promoting the production of energy from fat and sugar in the mitochondria, glucose removal from the bloodstream may be enhanced and insulin function improved.

Indeed, alpha-lipoic acid has been shown to decrease insulin resistance and is prescribed frequently in Europe as a treatment for peripheral neuropathy (nerve damage) associated with diabetes. In the United States, the American Diabetes Association has suggested that alpha-lipoic acid plus vitamin E may be helpful in combating some of the health complications associated with diabetes, including heart disease, vision problems, nerve damage, and kidney disease.

Although there have been relatively few studies conducted with alpha-lipoic acid in humans, it appears to be safe as a dietary supplement. Intakes of as much as 600 mg/day have been used for treatment of diabetic neuropathy, with no serious side effects. The most effective daily dose in these studies is 300–600 mg/day, but a 100 mg/day maintenance dose may more appropriate for more general antioxidant support and nerve protection.

GYMNEMA SYLVESTRE

Gymnema sylvestre is a plant used medicinally in India and Southeast Asia for treatment of "sweet urine," or what we refer to in the West as diabetes or hyperglycemia. In ancient Indian texts, gymnema is referred to as *gurmar*, which means "sugar killer" in Sanskrit. Gymnema leaves, whether extracted or infused into a tea, suppress glucose absorption and reduce the sensation of sweetness in foods—effects that may deliver important health benefits for individuals who want to lower their blood-sugar levels.

Gymnema sylvestre leaves contain gymnemic acids, which are known to suppress transport of glucose from the intestine into the bloodstream, and a small protein, gurmar, that can interact with receptors on the tongue to decrease the sensation of sweetness in many foods. Modern scientific methods have isolated at least nine different fractions of gymnemic acids that possess hypoglycemic activity. The effect of gymnema extract on lowering blood levels of glucose, cholesterol, and triglycerides is fairly gradual, typically taking a few days to several weeks. Very high doses of dried gymnema leaves may even help to repair the cellular damage that causes (and is caused by) excessive blood-sugar exposure.

Several human studies conducted on gymnema for treatment of diabetes have shown significant reduction in blood glucose, glycosylated hemoglobin (an index of blood-sugar control), and insulin requirements (allowing insulin therapy to be reduced). Gymnema appears to increase the effectiveness of insulin rather than causing the body to produce more —although the precise mechanism by which this occurs remains unknown.

At typical recommended doses (see below), dietary supplements containing gymnema are not associated with significant adverse side effects. Mild gastrointestinal upset may occur if gymnema is taken on an empty stomach, so consumption with meals is recommended. Caution is urged, however, with extremely high doses, which may have the potential to induce hypoglycemia (abnormally low blood sugar) in susceptible individuals.

Most human studies have been conducted in diabetic patients and have used 400 mg of gymnema extract per day, in conjunction with conventional oral antidiabetic medications, to lower blood glucose and reduce insulin requirements. In nondiabetics, smaller doses may be effective in helping to control blood-sugar and insulin fluctuations.

BANABA LEAF

Banaba leaf is a medicinal plant that grows in India, Southeast Asia, and the Philippines. Traditional uses include brewing tea from the leaves as a treatment for diabetes and hyperglycemia (elevated blood sugar). The hypoglycemic (blood-sugar-lowering) effect of banaba leaf extract is similar to that of insulin, which induces glucose transport from the blood into the cells.

Banaba leaf extract contains a triterpenoid compound known as corosolic acid, which has actions in stimulating glucose transport into cells. As such, banaba plays a role in regulating levels of glucose and insulin in the blood. For some people, fluctuations in blood sugar and insulin are related to appetite, hunger, and various food cravings—particularly cravings for carbohydrates such as bread and sweets. By keeping blood-sugar and insulin levels in check, banaba may be an effective supplement for controlling the glycation of collagen and elastin in skin.

The blood sugar–regulating properties of banaba have been demonstrated in cell-culture, animal, and human studies. In isolated cells, the active ingredient in banaba extract, corosolic acid, is known to stimulate glucose uptake. In diabetic mice, rats, and rabbits, banaba feeding reduces elevated blood-sugar and insulin levels to normal. In humans with type-II diabetes, banaba extract, at a dose of 16–48 mg per day for four to eight weeks, has been shown to be effective in reducing blood-sugar levels (5–30 percent reduction) and maintaining tighter control of blood-sugar fluctuations.

At suggested doses, 8–48 mg per day, no adverse side effects are expected from banaba extract. Higher doses should be avoided, however, to prevent the possible hypoglycemic effects (headache, dizziness, fatigue) commonly associated with extremely low blood-glucose levels.

BITTER MELON *(MOMORDICA CHARANTIA)*

Bitter melon (*Momordica charantia*) has been used traditionally in Asia and South America as a folk remedy for diabetes and other ailments. Several small studies of various bitter-melon juices and powders indicate that it may lower blood sugar in diabetic people.

PANAX (ASIAN) GINSENG

Panax (Asian) ginseng has been used as a folk remedy in China and Korea for over a thousand years. In addition to its effects in controlling cortisol as an adaptogen against stress (see Chapter 6), various studies on animals show that Asian ginseng can lower blood sugar, improve glucose utilization, and increase insulin production. A placebo-controlled clinical study showed that 100–200 mg of an Asian ginseng extract reduced hemoglobin glycosylation and improved glucose tolerance without side effects. The standard dose is 100–200 mg daily of extracts standardized to 4–7 percent ginsenosides.

FENUGREEK

Fenugreek is a well-known spice that has been used in Asia and Africa to treat various ailments, including diabetes. The active, blood sugar–lowering principles of fenugreek have not been entirely elucidated, but dietary fiber and saponins (which are also antioxidants) may contribute. Fenugreek seeds contain a high proportion (40 percent) of a soluble fiber known as mucilage. This fiber forms a gelatinous structure that may have effects on slowing the digestion and absorption of sugar from the intestine. Other studies suggest that it is not the fiber in fenugreek that accounts for its effects in controlling blood sugar, but rather an amino acid extracted from fenugreek seeds (4-hydroxyisoleucine) that may stimulate insulin secretion (direct beta-cell stimulation) and help control blood-sugar levels.

. . . .
.
.

CHAPTER 9

Supplements for the Control of Eicosanoids

As with other areas where we can use supplements to "rebalance" certain aspects of metabolism, the same is true of eicosanoids. Remember from previous chapters that eicosanoids are hormonelike cellular messengers that can be proinflammatory or anti-inflammatory in nature. Simply by eating more of the right types of fats (anti-inflammatory omega-3s) and fewer of the wrong type (proinflammatory omega-6s), we shift the balance away from "bad" eicosanoids and toward "good" eicosanoids, and in doing so, we reduce overall levels of inflammation throughout the body.

ESSENTIAL FATTY ACIDS

The term "essential fatty acids" refers to two fatty acids, linoleic acid and linolenic acid, that our bodies cannot synthesize and thus which must be consumed in the diet. (Vitamins and minerals are also termed "essential" because the human body cannot make them and therefore must consume them.) These essential fatty acids are needed for the production of compounds known as eicosanoids, which help regulate inflammation, blood clotting, blood pressure, heart rate, immune response, and a wide variety of other biological processes.

Linoleic acid is a polyunsaturated fatty acid with eighteen carbon atoms and two double bonds. It is considered an "omega-6," or "n-6," fatty acid because the first of its double bonds occurs at the sixth carbon from the omega end. It is also referred to as C18:2n6 (meaning eighteen carbons, two double bonds, with the first double bond at n-6 position). It is found in vegetable and nut oils such as sunflower, safflower, corn, soy, and peanut oil. Most Americans get adequate levels of these omega-6 oils in their diets, due to a high consumption of vegetable oil–based margarine, salad dressings, and mayonnaise.

Linolenic acid, or alpha-linolenic acid, is also an eighteen-carbon polyunsaturated fatty acid, but it is classified as an "omega-3," or "n-3," fatty acid because its first double bond (of three) is located at the third carbon from the omega end. It is also known as C18:3n3 (meaning eighteen carbons, three double bonds, with the first double bond at the n-3 position). Good dietary sources for linolenic acid are flaxseed oil (51 percent linolenic acid), soy oil (7 percent), walnuts (7 percent), and canola oil (9 percent), as well as margarine derived from canola oil. For example, a tablespoon of canola oil or canola oil margarine provides about 1 gram of linolenic acid.

If you think back to the original type of diet early humans relied upon for survival—the so-called caveman diet—it provided a much more balanced mix of n-3 and n-6 fatty acids. Over the last century, modern diets have come to rely heavily on fats derived from vegetable oils (n-6)—bringing the ratio of n-6 to n-3 fatty acids from the caveman's ratio of about 1:1 to the modern-day range of 20–30:1. The unbalanced intake of n-6 fatty acids (high) to n-3 fatty acids (low) sets the stage for increases in blood viscosity (and tendency of blood to clot), vasoconstriction (and elevated blood pressure), and inflammatory processes (involved in everything from heart health to pain levels). Yikes!

Fatty acids of the n-3 variety, however, have opposing biological effects to those of the n-6 fatty acids, meaning that a higher intake of n-3 oils can deliver anti-inflammatory, antithrombotic (clot-preventing), and vasodilatory (blood pressure–lowering) effects that can lead to benefits in terms of heart disease, hypertension, diabetes, and a wide variety of inflammatory conditions such as rheumatoid arthritis and ulcerative colitis.

In the body, linoleic acid (n-6) is metabolized to arachidonic acid, a precursor to specific "bad" eicosanoids that can promote vasoconstriction and elevated blood pressure. Linolenic acid (n-3), however, is metabolized in the body to EPA (eicosapentaenoic acid) and DHA (docosahexaenoic acid). EPA serves as the precursor to prostaglandin E3, which may have vasodilatory properties on blood vessels, effects that can counteract the vasoconstriction caused by n-6 fatty acids. DHA has been associated with optimal brain development in infants.

Recent studies have shown that the consumption of linolenic acid and other n-3 fatty acids offers wide-ranging anti-inflammatory benefits. This effect is thought to be mediated through the synthesis of EPA and DHA. Fish oils contain large amounts of both EPA and DHA, and the majority of studies in this area have used various concentrations of fish oil supplements to demonstrate the health benefits of these essential fatty acids. For example, 1 gram of menhaden oil (a common source) provides about 300 mg of these fatty acids. EPA is known to induce an antithrombotic (clot-preventing) effect through its inhibition of platelet cyclooxygenase (which converts arachidonic acid to thromboxane A2, two compounds that are highly inflammatory) and the "less sticky" platelets that result. Fish oil, with its high content of EPA and DHA, may also protect against heart disease through an anti-inflammatory effect (via reduced cytokine production and/or increased nitric oxide production in the endothelium).

There is also some evidence that omega-3 fatty acids from fish oil and flaxseed may help improve insulin sensitivity (thus reducing glycation) and reduce the perception of stress (thus decreasing cortisol exposure). A recent expert scientific advisory board at the National Institutes of Health highlighted the importance of a balanced intake of n-6 and n-3 fatty acids to reduce the adverse effects of elevated (inflammatory) arachidonic acid, a metabolic product of n-6 metabolism. The committee recommended a reduction in the intake of n-6 fatty acids (linoleic acid) and an increase in n-3 (linolenic acid, DHA, EPA) intake.

No serious adverse side effects should be expected from regular consumption of essential fatty acid supplements, whether from fish oil or other common oil supplements (see below). Due to the tendency of n-3 fatty acids to reduce platelet aggregation (i.e., "thin" the blood), increased bleeding times can occur in some individuals.

The best dietary sources of omega-3 fatty acids are fish such as trout, tuna, salmon, mackerel, herring, and sardines, which all contain about 1–2 grams of n-3 oils per three- or four-ounce serving. A minimum of 4–5 grams of linoleic acid (but no more than 6–7 grams) and 2–3 grams of linolenic acid are recommended per day. Supplements of linoleic acid (n-6) are typically not needed, whereas linolenic acid (n-3) supplements (4–10 g/day) and/or concentrated EPA/DHA supplements (400–1,000 mg/day) are recommended to support cardiovascular health. Total DHA/EPA intake should approach about 1 gram per day, evenly split between the two sources.

The most common supplemental source of essential fatty acids is fish oil—a good source of the omega-3 fatty acids. Other oils, such as flaxseed, borage seed, and evening primrose, are rich sources of essential fatty acids but typically do not provide the high levels of concentrated EPA/DHA found in many fish oil supplements. The highest-quality fish oil supplements should provide 18–30 percent EPA and 12–20 percent DHA. The higher the EPA/DHA content, the better (but also the more expensive).

EVENING PRIMROSE OIL

Evening primrose oil (EPO) is most commonly used for relieving inflammatory conditions associated with women's health, for example, premenstrual syndrome, fibrocystic breasts, and menopausal symptoms, such as hot flashes.

Sixty to 80 percent of evening primrose oil is the essential fatty acid linoleic acid. Gamma-linoleic acid (GLA) is synthesized by the body from linoleic acid and comprises 8–14 percent of the oil. GLA is a precursor of prostaglandin E1 (PGE1), a deficiency of which has been documented in some women with premenstrual syndrome (PMS) and cyclical breast pain. Since decreased levels of PGE1 can increase the pain-inducing effect of the hormone prolactin on breast tissue, it is thought that this may be a primary cause of many of the symptoms associated with PMS.

In addition to its applications for specific detrimental effects of the menstrual cycle, theories for non–gender related uses of evening primrose oil are prevalent. PGE1 has beneficial anti-inflammatory, antiplatelet, and vasodilating properties. Because essential fatty acids are claimed to have positive effects on certain skin diseases, supplementation with evening primrose oil could also alleviate eczema and dermatitis. In a double-blind crossover study of men taking either fish oil alone or fish oil plus evening primrose oil, the combination led to a significant 12 percent decrease in atherogenic (related to deterioration of artery walls) and inflammatory markers, whereas fish oil alone led to a 6 percent decrease in the same markers. Finally, evening primrose oil has been demonstrated to decrease platelet aggregation and atherosclerotic plaques, both associated with inflammatory pathways.

Evening primrose oil appears to be quite safe. Because it hinders platelet aggregation, EPO supplements may thin the blood and may increase the anticoagulant effect of drugs such as warfarin. The most common dose of evening primrose oil is

1–4 grams per day of a preparation containing approximately 10 percent GLA.

BORAGE OIL

Borage seeds are a rich source of a gamma-linolenic acid (GLA), whose medicinal properties have been demonstrated in areas such as anti-inflammatory activity, immune-system modulation, and management of atopic eczema (excessive proliferation of skin cells) and other skin maladies.

Borage seed oil typically contains 20–30 percent GLA, a naturally occurring polyunsaturated fatty acid of the omega-6 series. (GLA can also be found in evening primrose oil and black currant oil.) GLA favors the formation of anti-inflammatory and anticlotting precursors. Specifically, GLA is transformed in the human body as di-homo gamma linolenic acid (DGLA), which leads to the formation of the 1-series prostaglandins (PG1s) rather than the formation of the 2-series prostaglandins (PG2s). PG2s have proinflammatory and clotting properties. DGLA also suppresses the formation of 4-series leukotrienes, which are also proinflammatory.

Studies have shown that individuals with active rheumatoid arthritis, an inflammatory condition, experienced an improvement in their symptoms when they were given between 322 and 1,960 mg daily of GLA in the form of a borage oil supplement for six months. In another study, a subgroup of a larger sample population experienced some relief of their atopic eczema when taking 345 mg of GLA (1,500 mg borage oil) for twenty-four weeks. Other studies in humans and animals have shown the positive effect of GLA supplementation on the stimulation of white blood cells and on the promotion of anti-inflammatory metabolites.

Borage seed oil is generally considered safe. The freshness of the oil is important. The oil contains a significant amount of polyunsaturated fatty acids (i.e., GLA, alpha-linoleic acid, etc.) that could be damaged in the presence of oxygen (oxidation) and UV light. Under these conditions, the oil would become strong tasting and smelly (rancid). The presence of naturally occurring vitamin E (an antioxidant) can be found in the oil. Blending additional amounts of vitamin E or other antioxidants, such as vitamin C or rosemary, helps to keep the oil more stable. Borage seed oil should be kept refrigerated to slow the oxidative process. Recommended doses of GLA range from 100 to 300 mg per day (one tablespoon of the oil or one to three softgels daily). There may be variations between different brands, based on the extent of the oil extraction from the seed.

BOSWELLIA SERRATA

The boswellia plant produces a sap that has been used in traditional Indian medicine as a treatment for arthritis and inflammatory conditions. The primary compounds thought to be responsible for the anti-inflammatory activity of boswellia are known as boswellic acids, which are thought to interfere with enzymes that contribute to inflammation and pain.

The plant has a long history of safe and effective use as a mild anti-inflammatory to reduce pain and stiffness and promote increased mobility. It lacks many of the gastrointestinal side effects commonly reported for synthetic anti-inflammatory medications. A number of studies have shown that boswellic acids may possess anti-inflammatory activity at least as potent as common over-the-counter medications such as ibuprofen and aspirin. In one study of patients with rheumatoid arthritis, pain and swelling was reduced following three months of boswellia use. Although there are no reports of serious adverse side effects from taking boswellia, in some cases it may be associated with mild gastrointestinal upset (heartburn, after-taste, and nausea) and should therefore be taken with food.

The typical recommended dose of boswellia is 400–1,200 mg per day of an extract standardized to contain approximately 30–65 percent boswellic acids. The extract should be consumed in divided doses of 100–400 mg each for approximately two to three months to achieve benefits in terms of reduced pain and improved mobility.

BROMELAIN AND PAPAIN

The term "proteolytic" is a catchall term referring to enzymes that digest protein. Supplemental forms can incorporate any of a wide variety of enzymes, including trypsin, chymotrypsin, pancreatin, bromelain, papain, and a range of fungal proteases. In the body, proteolytic digestive enzymes are produced in the pancreas, but supplemental forms may come from fungal or bacterial sources, extraction from plants (such as papain from the papaya and bromelain from pineapples), or extraction from the pancreas of livestock animals (trypsin/chymotrypsin). The primary uses of proteolytic enzymes in dietary supplements are as digestive enzymes, anti-inflammatory agents, and pain relievers.

Perhaps the strongest evidence for benefits of proteolytic enzyme supplements come from numerous European studies showing various enzyme blends to be effective in accelerating recovery from exercise and injury in athletes, as well as improving tissue repair in patients following surgery. In one study of soccer players suffering from ankle injuries, proteolytic enzyme supplements accelerated healing and got players back on the field about 50 percent faster than athletes assigned to receive a placebo tablet. A handful of other small trials in athletes have shown that enzymes can help reduce inflammation, speed healing of bruises and other tissue injuries (including fractures), and reduce overall recovery time when compared to athletes taking a placebo. In patients recovering from facial and various reconstructive surgeries, treatment with proteolytic enzymes significantly reduced swelling, bruising, and stiffness compared to placebo groups. Similar findings have been reported for other painful or inflammatory conditions, including carpal tunnel syndrome, fibromyalgia, facial bruising, ankle sprains, muscle soreness, and others.

Proteolytic enzymes are generally considered to be quite safe, although mild gastrointestinal side effects (heartburn) may result in some individuals. People at risk for gastric or duodenal ulcers may want to avoid enzyme supplements that could aggravate ulcerated tissues. In addition, because proteolytic enzyme supplements also tend to produce a modest anticoagulant (blood-thinning) effect, they should probably not be used in conjunction with warfarin or other blood-thinning agents.

The dosage or "strength" of an enzyme supplement is typically expressed in "activity units" that refer to the enzyme's ability to digest a certain amount of protein. Because the same milligram amount of a particular enzyme may have different activity units based on its processing and blending, it may be advisable to select an enzyme supplement that employs a combination of enzymes that show activity at different pH levels. Also, look for a brand that is "enteric coated"—meaning that the formulation is protected from early digestion in the stomach in order to provide optimal delivery of the enzymes to the intestines, where they can perform their actions.

FLAXSEED OIL

Flaxseed is just what it sounds like—the seed of the flax plant. The typical use of flaxseed is as a source of the essential fatty acids linolenic acid (LN, an omega-3) and linoleic acid (LA, an omega-6). Flaxseed oil is about 57 percent LN and about 17 percent LA. As described above, LN can be converted into decosahexaenoic acid (DHA) and eicosapentaenoic acid (EPA), fatty acids that are precursors to anti-inflammatory and anti-atherogenic prostaglandins.

Regular flaxseed consumption has been associated with improvements in the ratio of omega-3 to omega-6 fatty acids in the blood, which may offer protection from atherogenesis and relief from inflammatory conditions. A number of animal studies have shown a beneficial role of flaxseed oil in delaying breast cancer progression and preventing colon cancer, sometimes as much as a 50 percent reduction compared to control groups not fed flaxseed. A clear and consistent reduction in proinflammatory markers (e.g., tumor necrosis factor and interleukin) has been noted in human subjects supplemented with flaxseed oil.

Effective multigram doses of flaxseed or flaxseed oil are unlikely to pose any adverse side effects. A note of caution is warranted, however, in cases of comprised blood clotting, such as hemophilia or liver disease, due to the tendency of flaxseed to reduce platelet aggregation and prolong bleeding times. A similar cautionary note is advisable for individuals undergoing surgical procedures, which may predispose the patient to excessive bleeding.

Beneficial effects have been observed at daily doses of 30–40 grams (2–4 ounces) of either concentrated flaxseed oil or whole/ground flaxseeds. Popular uses for the oil include salad dressings and spreads; the seeds are often used in baked goods or sprinkled on cereal or other foods.

GINGER *(ZINGIBER OFFICINALE)*

Ginger has been used throughout history as an aid for many gastrointestinal disturbances as well as to relieve inflamed joints. The most active chemical compounds in ginger are known as the gingerols, which are also the most aromatic compounds in this root and which are thought to be the reason why ginger can inhibit substances that cause the pain and inflammation associated with osteoarthritis. For example, in osteoarthritis patients taking powdered ginger, 75 percent of the subjects reported decreased pain and swelling. There are no reported adverse effects of taking ginger, and it does not have any reported interactions with medications. Most studies have used 1 gram of powdered, dried ginger root per day.

WHITE WILLOW BARK

The bark of the white willow tree is a source of salicin and other salicylates, compounds that are similar in structure to aspirin (acetyl salicylic acid). Salicin, which is the primary active compound in white willow bark and which can be converted in the body into salicylic acid, has powerful effects as an anti-inflammatory and pain reliever. Native Americans are thought to have used ground willow bark and bark steeped for tea as a medicinal remedy for everything from pain to fevers. Until synthetic aspirin could be produce in large quantities, white willow bark was the treatment of choice for reducing fevers, relieving headache and arthritis pain, and controlling swelling. Today, white willow bark is often used as a natural alternative to aspirin. Although synthetic aspirin is clearly a more effective pain reliever and anti-inflammatory agent compared to the weaker bark extract, white willow can also serve as a source of tannins, a combination that may provide a synergistic action with regard to antioxidant effects (tannins are a class of polyphenols; see Chapter 7).

Stomach ulcers and other gastrointestinal complaints such as nausea and diarrhea are common side effects from prolonged high-dose consumption of either synthetic aspirin or white willow bark extracts—but lower, maintenance doses of the natural bark extract are often tolerated much better than the more powerful synthetic aspirin. Individuals with concerns about blood clotting and bleeding time should use aspirin and white willow with caution, as both have the potential to interfere with platelet aggregation and to prolong bleeding time (i.e., create a "blood-thinning" effect).

For those looking for a "gentler" approach to balancing inflammation management, low-dose white willow may be an effective alternative to aspirin. Standardized extracts of white willow bark are available. Total salicin intake is typically 25–100 mg per day for promoting inflammatory balance.

. . . .
                ·
                ·

CHAPTER 10

The FACE Program:
A Closer Look

Dwell in possibility.

— Emily Dickinson
American poet, 1830–1886

At this point, you have all of the information you need to put the FACE program into action in your daily life. By now, you already understand the "why" of using diet, exercise, and supplements to modulate these four important aspects of skin metabolism. Now comes the "how" of putting the program into practice—and it couldn't be easier.

THE "FACE" PROGRAM: STEP 1

Each day, you'll want to perform some type of exercise or stress management, such as meditation or yoga. Both will control cortisol levels, but physical activity will also modulate blood-sugar levels and exposure to free radicals and eicosanoids.

For more information on how exercise benefits the skin, refer back to the section entitled "Exercise Your Skin" in Chapter 3. Also, Appendix B at the back of the book outlines an easy-to-follow exercise program that will help you to increase your systemic circulation.

THE "FACE" PROGRAM: STEP 2

At every meal, you'll want to follow the "Helping Hand" approach to eating, so that each time you eat, you're consuming a balanced blend of carbohydrates, protein, and fats. For more information on this step, refer back to the section entitled "The Helping Hand Diet" in Chapter 5. Also, try some of the delicious recipes included in Appendix A. Each is balanced according to the metabolic control principles that I advocate with the FACE program (see Chapters 6 through 9).

THE "FACE" PROGRAM: STEP 3

Select a supplement regimen to address one or more of the aspects of metabolic control as outlined in the FACE program.

Using the FACE Program to Prevent, Reduce, or Eliminate Wrinkles

If you are most concerned about **wrinkles,** then a regimen focused on *cortisol control* (the first step in wrinkle development) and *glycation control* (the second step in wrinkle development) should be your objective. This means selecting one or more supplements from Chapter 6 ("Supplements for Control of Cortisol") and a supplement from Chapter 8 ("Supplements for Control of AGEs"). You may also want to select one of the "adaptogenic" supplements known to control *both* cortisol and blood sugar, such as ginseng or cordyceps. (See "Summary of Supplements," below.)

Using the FACE Program to Prevent or Treat Acne

If **acne** treatment and prevention is your main concern, then you'll want to focus your supplement choices mostly toward *cortisol control* (to reduce oil overproduction) and also toward *control of free-radical damage* (Chapter 7, "Supplements for Control of Oxidation") and *control of eicosanoid-induced inflammation* (Chapter 9, "Supplements for Control of Eicosanoids"). (Also, see summary of supplements, below.)

Using the FACE Program to Deal with "Problem Skin"

If your concern is generalized "problem skin," such as **rosacea, dermatitis,** or **eczema,** you will want to focus your supplement regimen on *controlling cortisol* (Chapter 6, "Supplements for Control of Cortisol") and *controlling inflammation* (Chapter 9, "Supplements for Control of Eicosanoids"). There is less need to focus on free-radical modulation or blood-sugar control. (See "Summary of Supplements," below.)

Summary of Supplements
For Controlling Cortisol (Chapter 6)

- Beta-sitosterol
- Damiana
- *Rhodiola rosea*
- Valerian
- Epimedium
- Ginseng
- Schisandra
- Theanine
- Ashwagandha *(Withania somnifera)*
- Cordyceps *(Cordyceps sinensis)*
- Magnolia bark *(Magnolia officinalis)*
- Kava kava *(Piper methysticum)*
- Passionflower *(Passiflora incarnata)*

For Controlling Free-Radical Damage (Chapter 7)

- Antioxidants
- Spirulina
- Beta-carotene
- Lycopene
- Vitamin A
- Vitamin C (ascorbic acid)
- Flavonids/polyphenols
- Lutein/zeaxanthin
- Vitamin E (tocopherols and tocotrienols)
- Green tea *(Camellia sinensis)*
- Gotu kola *(Centella asiatica)*

For Controlling AGEs (Chapter 8)

- Chromium
- Zinc
- *Gymnema sylvestre*
- Panax (Asian) ginseng
- Bitter melon (*Momordica charantia*)
- Vanadium
- Alpha-lipoic acid
- Banaba leaf
- Fenugreek

For Controlling Eicosanoid-Induced Inflammation (Chapter 9)

- Linoleic acid
- Borage oil
- Bromelain and papain
- White willow bark
- Evening primrose oil
- *Boswellia serrata*
- Flaxseed oil
- Ginger (*Zingiber officinale*)

THE "FACE" PROGRAM: STEP 4

Visit www.cortisolconnection.com to let me know how you're doing and to receive updated scientific information as well as specific recommendations for topical cosmetics and dietary supplements.

Let's take another look at how the various factors addressed by the FACE program interact (Figure 10.1).

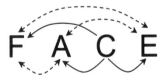

Figure 10.1

It is vitally important to keep the interrelated nature of metabolic control in mind. The most effective regimen for promoting skin function, health, and appearance is a multi-faceted one that simultaneously addresses as many aspects of metabolism as possible.

. . . .
                  .
                  .
                  .

CHAPTER 11

Putting It All Together: Becoming Comfortable in Your Own Skin

Beauty is not in the face; beauty is a light in the heart.

— Kahlil Gibran
Lebanese-American writer, 1883–1931

This final chapter will help you make all this know-how work on a more than skin-deep basis. So far you have learned about the inner culprits that cause damage to the skin and how using the FACE program can remedy that damage and keep you looking—and feeling—youthful, fresh, and radiant. Now it's time to invite some of the experts who specialize in natural skin care to speak about facial beauty from the inside out. If you follow the FACE program and take the best of what these experts have to say as it applies to you, you will have a beauty-care regimen that fits who you are, nourishes your health and entire being, and allows your natural beauty to shine forth radiantly—no matter what your age is.

YOUR SKIN
A REFLECTION OF YOUR INNER BEING

Making women's faces look beautiful is an industry that has existed for thousands of years. In modern times, this industry has become large, mostly corporate, and based on particular standards of beauty that can cause women to feel as though they require a makeover, a face-lift, or a cabinet full of facial creams to elevate them to the current standards of beauty. This pressure to make yourself into something other than what you are has touched even the most independent, intelligent women, many of whom spend copious amounts of time and money trying to "get it right." Even women who have decided to sidestep this insistent invitation often secretly feel that they are missing something in terms of beauty.

We were fortunate to locate several skin-care experts who don't see things this way at all. Instead, their perspective is helping women be as healthy, as natural, and as balanced as they can be. In their work as aestheticians, product developers, facial acupuncturists, and dermatologists, they seek to nourish the whole human being by means of nourishing the skin. As you read what these experts have to say in these pages, you will discover how you want to use your skin-care regimen as a way to care for your entire being. This makes the prospect of caring for your skin much more than another habit to begin or improve; it opens the door to caring for yourself in a much more accepting and conscious way and will lead to healing your heart and soul as you heal your skin.

Let's hear what our experts have to say. First we'll introduce each one to you. Next, we'll see what they all agree on. Then, we'll explore their *different* points of view on a given skin-related subject. And, finally, we'll present each expert's unique perspective. Read the following sections with an open mind to see which ways might work best for you:

OUR PANEL OF SKIN-CARE EXPERTS

To give you a good range of expertise from professionals on different parts of the skin-care spectrum, so that you can benefit from their knowledge and wisdom and apply these fruits (sometimes literally!) to your own face, we interviewed the following people:

Marianne Damhuis: Aethestician

Originally from the Netherlands, Marianne Damhuis is an aesthetician in private practice in Sausalito, California, who uses a natural approach to skin care. A radiant-looking woman in her fifties who practices what she preaches in terms of a lifestyle that promotes beautiful skin, she brings her spiritual life to her work and believes that you can do the same.

Shelley Rosenfeld: Licensed Aesthetician

As the name of her business, Conscious Skin and Body Care (Alameda, California), implies, Shelley sees herself as a wellness educator, helping to demystify some unfortunate skin-care myths and promoting facial beauty as an outgrowth of knowledgeable self-care and the most natural approaches. An expert aesthetician at a world-renowned spa in Northern California before becoming a business owner, she has had extensive advanced training at the International Dermal Institute, and she continually studies to enhance her skills as a skin- and body-care therapist.

Elina Fedotova: Holistic Practitioner, Cosmetic Chemist, Medical Aesthetician, and Creator of Elina Elite Skin Care Collection

Elina makes by hand an all-natural skin-care product line containing organic fruits, vegetables, herbs, vitamins, essential oils, and other natural ingredients. Her products are endorsed and distributed by doctors, aestheticians, and plastic surgeons throughout the world. Originally from Russia, Elina has salons in Kalamazoo, Michigan, and Chicago, Illinois.

John Nieters: Licensed Acupuncturist

John Nieters, L.Ac., is an acupuncturist in Alameda, California. Specializing in internal medicine, he also does cosmetic, or facial, acupuncture. Extensively trained in Chinese medicine, John has an M.S. in traditional Chinese medicine, is board certified as a Diplomate through the National Board of Acupuncture Orthopedics, holds a national certification in Chinese herbal medicine, and teaches Chinese nutrition and herbal medicine at the Academy of Chinese Culture and Health Science in Oakland, California. He hosts a call-in radio show based in San Francisco called *The Balancing Point* (Thursday mornings from 8:00–9:00 A.M. on KEST 1450 AM).

Karen Burke, M.D., Ph.D.: Dermatologist and Research Scientist

A dermatologist and research scientist in private practice in New York City, Karen is on staff at Mt. Sinai Medical Center, Department of Dermatology. With extensive research in antioxidants and a Ph.D. in biophysics, she is an expert on the effects of vitamins and supplements on skin. She is known for her research on the prevention and reversal of aging of the skin, as well the prevention and treatment of skin cancer. A focus of her work has been demonstrating the efficacy of topical and oral antioxidants in reversing photoaging of the skin and preventing skin cancer. A member of many organizations, including the American Academy of Dermatology and the American Medical Association, she has been a consultant to many corporations and has authored numerous articles as well as four books: *Great Skin for Life, Thin Thighs, Thin Thighs for Life,* and *Thin Thighs Diet and Workout* (Octopus).

Contact information for each of these experts is listed in the Resources section, located at the back of the book.

WHAT THE EXPERTS AGREE ON

All our experts agree that the FACE program's elements are important in caring for the skin. They agree that for good, healthy, radiant skin, controlling cortisol is essential. Equally important, they also believe, is the establishment of a balanced, wholesome diet; the use of supplements; exercise; and a lifestyle that involves as little stress as possible.

Controlling Stress

SHELLEY "Stress raises the cortisol level, raising the inflammation level, which shows up in the skin. They say inflammation is the start of all diseases. When the skin is red, that means *all* the cells in the body are red. Inflammation in the skin means there's inflammation in the cells." The causes? "Lifestyle. Genetics. Sun damage. Consuming inflammatory foods, such as caffeine and certain spices. We can have an inflammatory *lifestyle*, due to constant stress." The solution? "The main way to address inflammation is through diet, exercise, meditation, whatever; we must cut down on the use of caffeine and alcohol.

"What goes into aging gracefully? Exercising. Eating right. Doing things that relieve stress. Taking care of the skin. Drinking a lot of water and trying to live as stress-free as possible."

ELINA "Cortisol intoxicates the whole body. The skin, as the largest organ of the body, reacts to this intoxication. After being stressed, people commonly develop skin rashes. Almost all skin problems have a connection with stress and with overproduction of yeast in the body (e.g., candida).

"That's why the skin regimen should be natural. It should not cause stress by itself [by the presence of different toxic chemicals in the cosmetic products]. It should give a nourishing effect. A natural skin regimen must have anti-inflammatory effects; it must include antioxidants so it can restore damaged, oxidized cells on a cellular level and help to regenerate the skin."

Skin problems can be addressed by taking a significant amount of antioxidants internally, eating a good healthy diet, and reducing stress in your life. "Every time you have stress, you're intoxicating your cells and creating the oxidation reaction, which produces free radicals. You need more antioxidants following stressful periods, in order to restore the system. So if you're taking lots of antioxidants, you're helping your whole body—including your skin—to recover from previous stress and free-radical damage, including your skin. So, for example, if you have lots of pigment spots and you're taking lots of anti-oxidants *internally* and using beneficial transdermal skin-care products, which have lots of antioxidants, *on* the skin, you are working that problem from both the inside-out and from the outside-in!"

Diet

MARIANNE "For different skin conditions, diet definitely makes a difference." She recommends fresh fruits and vegetables. "Whole foods, organic foods are the best," she emphasizes, "because they're healthy for the skin. Sometimes you detox through the skin."

SHELLEY recommends drinking plenty of fluids—water, juices, herbal teas, lemonade made from water and lemons (go easy on the sugar). "They flush away toxins and impurities. Eat high–water content foods, like grapes. Dehydration usually shows up last in our skin, because the inner organs need fluids first. Hydrated skin looks great, on the face and everywhere else!" (See "On Hydration," below, for more detail.)

ELINA cautions, "Watch what you eat. Sweets and caffeine aren't good for your overall health—or your face. Think lemonade (made from water, lemons, and minimal sugar) and herbal tea, not pop. Hot spicy foods and yeast-rich products can also lead to hormonal imbalance, and that shows up on your face. Eating vegetables is an essential part of true beauty."

JOHN includes a nutritional consultation when he first meets with his facial acupuncture patients. "I teach them Western nutrition and Chinese medical nutrition to get people to change their internal chemistry." As far as specific foods go, he says, "Shawn [the author of this book] and I probably agree on 98 percent of it."

On the plus side (foods to eat), John recommends:

1. "Brightly colored foods with high beta-carotene content and, ultimately, big vitamin A precursors, which are critical to the skin. They have all the antioxidants. Add as many of these as you can."

2. Omega-3 fatty acids, either from liquid cod-liver oil or fish oil, or by eating fatty fish or high-quality meat.

John recommends the liquid form of fish oil or cod-liver oil to almost all his patients: "The cod-liver oil and fish oil are the easiest sources for people. Cod-liver oil has high levels of vitamin A and vitamin D in it, which are very powerful for the body." He believes that *the single thing that makes the biggest difference is high quantities of high-quality omega-3 fatty acids*, because they're so anti-inflammatory and critical for the skin and health in general. We can live without simple carbohydrates in our diets, and we get way more protein than we need, even in the simplest vegetarian diet. But we need those good-quality fats to live, especially to provide for healthier skin."

Eating fatty fish or very high quality meat also provides good sources of omega-3 fatty acids. "Also, use meat from free-range cattle that's grass fed, bison that's grass fed, lamb, or wild game. Animals that eat grass convert the fatty acids to high levels of omega-3s. Once an animal has been on a feedlot for ninety days, it doesn't have any long-chain omega-3 fatty acids left, which makes this type of meat very inflammatory. So fish oil is the easiest way, if you're going to take a supplement, though it's much better to go out and have a bison burger or a piece of salmon."

Supplements

MARIANNE believes in supplements, "especially as you get older." She favors oils in particular, such as flaxseed oil and olive oil. "These oils are very good for the skin because they make the skin very moist." As to which supplements to take, she suggests, "All the supplements that you would take for your immune system and for your health, such as vitamin C and vitamin E."

SHELLEY advocates antioxidants: zinc for acne, grape seed extract for brown spots and pigmentation, willow bark for the salicylic acid, and the digestive enzymes propain and bromelain.

ELINA puts antioxidants into her topical products. "Discoloration of the skin is due to oxidation. It's the result of sun damage, of ultraviolet damage in the cells," she explains. "When people take more antioxidants internally, it helps them to regenerate and restore all the cells, including skin cells." She also suggests taking horse chestnut daily, to make veins and capillaries more flexible and supple.

Lifestyle
Being Relaxed
MARIANNE is very much in favor of including "oxygenation and deep breathing, like yoga, or total relaxation with long, deep breathing. Taking care of your circulation, so that you do slow exercises that really go into deep relaxation states. A lot of stretching and walking, yoga-type exercises. This is fabulous for the skin and certainly helps with stress reduction. A lot of people look so much younger than they are because of this."

JOHN views being relaxed as a key element of acupuncture: "When people go into that very relaxed state, they generally go into an alpha brain-wave state, which we all should go into regularly but tend not to. I tell people, 'This is just a way of reminding your body what it's supposed to be doing.' The important thing is to keep doing that all the time: 'Right now, on the bus—breathe!'"

Rhythm and Routine
SHELLEY "It's not about quick fixes, like going to get face lifts, but taking care of our whole being, and that includes our skin.

Create a regular rhythm of normal lifestyle habits. The body loves routine. Rise at about the same time each day, eat at about the same times each day, get adequate sleep about the same time of night, exercise at about the same times during the week—and so on."

Attitude and Peace of Mind

ELINA "I deal with so many people. Some do not have a difficult life, and yet they're so stressed, and others have an extremely challenging life but are not stressed. It depends on how you handle life.

"One client comes to the salon and says, 'I'm so stressed! I want to get my massage! Then my pedicure! Then my manicure! Now I'm doing a facial, then tomorrow we're going for a vacation!' And another client is a single mother with five children, working three jobs, saying, 'Oh, it's so relaxing, now. I finally got here. We're doing fine. My child is not sick anymore, and another one improved her grades. We're keeping things under control.' It's an absolutely different approach to life. It doesn't matter how stressful one life is and how not stressful another life is. It's how you're taking it and how you're controlling that stress."

Exercise

MARIANNE recommends a balance of relaxation and high-energy movement. In addition to doing slowing-down movements like stretching and yoga, "get your circulation going by doing high-energy exercise, such as brisk walking, dancing, trampoline, or something else that revs up your system. And exercise is really important for the emotions too, for mental health."

Elimination

MARIANNE advocates colonics and cleansers. "I feel so good when I do it. I think it does keep you healthy to keep your colon clean. [It's also important] to watch your food."

SHELLEY recommends brushing the skin. "Use a loofah or body brush to rev circulation and clear cell debris from the epidermis. Light saunas and hot (not too hot) herbal baths also are great for helping skin excrete wastes." In addition, be sure to have regular and complete bowel movements.

ELINA believes that all skin problems "are related to intoxication. Not only do we manifest internal problems through the skin, but we can also eliminate toxins through the skin, such as with sweats. If we're less toxic inside, we'll have fewer skin-care problems. Burdock root tea and dandelion root tea are very classical formulas. You may go to the bathroom more and sweat more in the beginning, but you'll eliminate lots of toxins."

WHERE THE EXPERTS DIFFER

In this section, our experts put forth different opinions regarding diet, hydration, supplements, sunscreens, the treatment of certain skin conditions, cosmetic surgery, and when a visit to a dermatologist might be in order.

On Diet
What Not *to Eat*
MARIANNE "There are things that some people are allergic to—for example, alcohol or wheat or a lot of salt. It comes out in the skin; you can see it in the face. They may blow up or get dark circles under the eyes. It depends on their constitution."

SHELLEY cautions avoiding or at least minimizing known toxins and irritants such as carbonated drinks, coffee, and other stimulants; the "white poisons" of refined sugar and flour; fried foods (oil that's heated over 118° F is rancid); processed foods (choose real, whole foods found in nature); concentrates, such as juices (irritating to the stomach; dilute with water); chemical additives.

JOHN says, "Decrease amounts of sugars, particularly high-fructose corn syrup, but also anything that's really a simple carbohydrate. Because when you overload the body, you get a very rapid insulin response. And with that rapid insulin response, the body creates inflammation. So that inflammation is actually quite problematic.

"Simple carbohydrates mean, in particular, bread, pasta, etc. [note that carbohydrates can be a double-problem for many people, because wheat-based carbs can also be an allergen]. *Anything* that you're allergic to will create inflammation in the body. That's what an allergy is—an inflammatory response. For many people, wheat is not a problem, but for a relatively high percentage, it is and will cause inflammation. It will make the skin age faster."

What's Good to Eat

SHELLEY favors drinking "lots of unsweetened herbal teas, low-sodium soup broths, diluted juices, and purified water (not distilled), preferably with the minerals/electrolytes intact. Eat plenty of green vegetables for fiber, mostly raw, but steamed are okay."

JOHN advocates butter, if you feel you have to eat bread. "The simpler and more isolated the carbohydrate is, the more of a problem it is. If you just have bread by itself, it's more of a problem than having bread with butter on it. The butter is beneficial for a variety of reasons, one of which is that the fat will digest more slowly and will buffer the digestion of this high-carbohydrate food, so you won't have quite as rapid a rise in insulin. All these absurd dietary ideas that came along— 'Don't eat eggs; if you have toast, eat dry toast'—there's no science behind it. Try to lower the amount of unmodulated simple carbohydrates going into the system. If you're going to have toast, it's not quite as bad if you're having it with an omelet, because the protein in the fat will take longer to digest, so it will even out the sugar response."

On Hydration

ELINA agrees that drinking water is good, and she thinks that drinking herbal tea is even better. "For acne and inflammation on the skin, I think it's more beneficial to drink chamomile tea, calendula tea, or burdock root tea. Chamomile is healing and anti-inflammatory; plus, it's calming, reducing cortisol levels. Calendula has the same properties; also, it has very deep healing properties. [A combination of] burdock root and dandelion root is a very detoxing tea. Dandelion root is a very good hormonal-balancing and anti-inflammatory tea for people with acne and inflammatory problems. If you're taking these herbs in supplement form already, you can drink pure water. But I like to brew a tea. It tastes better." This is very traditional in Russia: "Every home has its own herbal teas. Not only in Russia, it's everywhere in Europe. The American Indians had it too. I think when the American people came and organized the new world, it was a great thing they did it, but I think they cut a lot of historical roots in traditional healing. They forgot how to do that, and are thinking that Tylenol can heal them, when a little chicken soup would be better."

On Supplements

MARIANNE agrees that it's important to take "a good antioxidant," yet she thinks it's hard to know just which supplements to take for your skin. "We're now hearing bad stuff about soy. And, they say that flaxseed oil isn't that well absorbed by the body. So it's very confusing." She sometimes takes chlorophyll, "because that oxygenates the whole system. So do leafy greens; I take a green supplement as well. But I'm in my fifties. When you're younger, you may not need as much. When you get older, I think you do need more. I recommend a good green supplement, an antioxidant, and oils."

She thinks it's up to the individual to determine what vitamins and supplements to take. And while she's in favor of nutritional supplements for good health, she advises, "I don't think that they're everything. If you just take supplements, and you're not eating right, I don't think you can just live on that. We have to keep everything working, and that includes a lot of things."

She adds, "Supplements are not totally harmless. I think there are areas where if you're on certain medication, they may counteract the medication or the medication may counteract the supplements. I think there are chemical reactions to supplements. You can't take supplements if you're doing certain medical treatments. I would check with a doctor."

KAREN recommends the following for controlling oxidation:

VITAMIN A: (not taken internally, but rather applied to the skin) While it's true that if you have too little vitamin A you get bad skin, you'd have to be really deficient, and that's very, very unlikely. I don't think we've ever seen a case of vitamin A deficiency in our society. She advises taking it internally only with reservations: "Too much is no good, especially during pregnancy."

However, putting it *on* the skin is good. Retinoic acid is one of the best things you can put on your skin to prevent aging. If you put on a high concentration, it makes your skin flaky and red. But you don't have to suffer those effects to reverse photoaging. You can reverse photoaging with a lower concentration by doing it regularly.

VITAMIN C: The minimum daily requirement is 50 mg, but some people can do well on as much as 3,000 mg/day.

VITAMIN E: Take the d-alpha-tocopherol succinate, not the synthetic kind. Take a total of 400 international units per day (the equivalent of 5,260 calories of sunflower oil).

SPIRULINA: I've never heard of it as an antioxidant, but it's a complete source of protein. It has all the essential amino acids. This is particularly valuable for vegetarians. If you're a vegetarian, you have to be sure to eat rice *and* beans, because one of them is missing the methionine and the other is missing the lysine. If you eat just rice and no beans and no meat, then you're missing one essential amino acid and you'd have a kind of protein deficiency.

BETA-CAROTENE: The body can make its own vitamin A out of beta-carotene.

LYCOPENE: I'm all for lycopene. I think it helps your health.

On Sunscreen

MARIANNE has a nuanced guidance to offer. On one hand, "I see a lot of damage from sun in my work. I think generally sunscreen is good to use. Wear a hat. Don't be exposed to lots and lots of sun." On the other hand, she feels it's good to "stay in the sun a little bit without any protection—just for little bit, to be balanced." She sees it as an individual decision. For herself, "I can intuitively tell how it feels—what's okay, or when it feels okay or not. I definitely think the sun, without some sun protection, is good for a little bit of time. It's like a sun bath, the same as an air bath or a water bath or a shower."

SHELLEY believes that "Everyone needs sunblock. Even if you have darker skin, you still need sunblock. There's still inflammation in the cells if you get sunburned." She advises using a sunscreen that contains zinc and titanium dioxide (iron oxide) as the main ingredients. "You can't just go outside all day with one application of sunblock; you have to reapply it. To figure out how often, take the amount of time it takes you to burn without anything on and multiply that by the SPF number. That's how long a single application will give you coverage. You can find natural sunblock products in the health food store."

She cautions against using sunscreens containing artificial colors and fragrances because they make you more sensitive to the effects of sunlight.

ELINA advises using "a minimum of SPF 15 sunscreen, every day. Even if you're not going out in the sun, protect yourself from reflection and lights."

She notes that the combination of overexposure to ultraviolet rays, eating trans-fat foods ("those hydrogenated oils"), plus being light complexioned, can cause skin cancers. "If you've experienced any cancer, even a cancer that is not dangerous, you need to eat tons of antioxidants and organically grown fruits and vegetables; avoid any kinds of trans-fats and animal protein; and use my skin-care products, with my sun-shelter makeup moisturizer, which has over 10 percent zinc and natural sunblock."

KAREN believes unequivocally that everyone needs sunscreen. "Put on as much as possible. You have to put it on every four hours to get the sunscreen effect, because every one and a half hours you perspire it off." Certain nutrients taken orally provide some ongoing protection: "If you take vitamin C (3,000 mg), vitamin E (4,000 mg), and selenium, you already have a little bit of a sunscreen effect and an SPF of about two or three all the time, so you don't have to put sunscreen on every hour and a half. And then any sunscreen you put on would add to the SPF. Take antioxidants to decrease the effect of sun damage, too."

She adds, "But there's no doubt that you need sunscreen. It makes you look old and wrinkled to have skin damage, and it gives skin cancer, the most common cancer. [Of all the cancers] melanoma is the biggest killer of young men and women under thirty. Some skin cancers aren't so invasive; some are just like a little mole—you get them cut off if you catch it early.

"Everyone needs frequently applied sunscreen. In the lab, when we measure the SPF, we apply a layer of lotion two millimeters thick and don't rub it in. But in real life people use much less, so an SPF 30 may only provide an SPF 15 or less. Wearing a low SPF is like riding a motorbike without any clothes on. No matter what factor you use, you should apply it twenty minutes before going out into the sun and reapply every ninety minutes. To cover your entire body, you'll need thirty milliliters of lotion—that's two good tablespoons—every ninety minutes. For a two-week holiday, you'll need at least six bottles of sunscreen. Lotion should sit on your skin as an active barrier; if it has been absorbed into your skin, it's not going to be as effective."

However, most effects of sun exposure are reversible. "In the short term, use a soothing after-sun product or an aloe vera cream. Take aspirin every four hours, or a natural vitamin E supplement to reduce the inflammation. If you have serious pain and blistering, see a doctor. In the long term, vitamins A and C, used often and in high doses, reverse the effects of sun damage. You might want to try a cream containing vitamin E (tocopherol) to soothe sunburned skin." One study showed that selenomethionine, a natural amino acid, reduces the skin damage caused by sunburn when applied to the skin and taken orally. Karen recommends taking 100 micrograms a day during the summer months, and 200 micrograms a day if you have a family history of cancer.

On Specific Skin Conditions
Acne

MARIANNE "Acne is very hard on the self-esteem. I think it's all about taking care of yourself and accepting yourself. And accepting that everything that happens passes. It's like weather.

So you get an outbreak in your skin, but you just take it the best you can and it will pass. People think that if you have two spots on your face, life is over—but other people are really looking at your eyes and your energy. When we look at a person we feel the energy, whether we're conscious of it or not. That's what people see, and that's what's important."

Still, "Keep away from things like caffeine and chocolate, any greasy foods, and fried foods."

SHELLEY "Acne is inflammation. Often, it's toxic buildup in the lymph system. Genetically, it's a weakness in the hair follicles. When acne is red and inflamed, there's infection underneath the skin and a lack of oxygen." When a client comes to see her because of acne, she'll calm the skin down but won't necessarily dry it out: "There needs to be that balance of oil and hydration on the skin."

To drain the lymph, Shelley cleans the skin well with a cleanser and a vacuum tool. She begins by exfoliating the skin with a salicylic peel made from willow bark. "What I'm doing is preparing the skin for the extraction, softening the oil." Then she extracts the blackheads by hand, using high-frequency antibacterial equipment. "I don't touch them if they are red," she notes, "because they're infected; that would spread the infection." Then she applies a calming masque and an oil-control formula. "I use no artificial fragrances or colors. That's very irritating to skin." At the end of the session, "I educate my clients to take care of their skin at home."

Shelley provides the following tips:

- If you're acne prone, avoid iodine and kelp in your multivitamins.

- Don't pick acne; it can spread the infection.

- Use anti-inflammatory products to clear up the bacteria, take zinc, and let it heal on its own. Avoid products that dry out the skin, like Clearasil or alcohol. Salicylic acid, an ingredient in some over-the-counter products, is good.

ELINA finds that some people never outgrow acne, but it does diminish over time. She recommends using her Oil Control Formula "to stop acne before it starts." Her product line includes an anti-inflammatory for acne and rosacea, "because acne and rosacea are usually inflammatory conditions of the skin as a result of hormonal imbalance."

Dry Skin

MARIANNE suggests, "For younger people—or for dry skin—I'd say use oils and that kind of supplement."

Dull Skin

SHELLEY explains, "As we get older, our dead skin cells slough off more and more slowly, so that's why skin gets dull-looking. When you get a facial, you're getting the dead skin cells off faster. When a dead skin cell comes off, a new one is born."

Rosacea

MARIANNE "If you have rosacea, keep away from caffeine, alcohol, spices."

SHELLEY describes rosacea as an inflammation, noting "the redness in the cheeks and nose. 'Rosacea' is a loose term referring to the redness. Redness can come from thin capillary walls." What to do: "Anti-inflammatory stuff is good. Eat cooling foods, like cucumbers, broccoli." What to avoid: "Alcohol, caffeine, spicy foods. Avoid hot water; don't put your face in the stream of the shower; avoid hot tubs, saunas."

ELINA "The most common inflammations of the skin, like rosacea and some dermatitis, all have similar issues. It's a hormonal imbalance, and I have a special cleanser and special toner for that."

Pigment Spots

ELINA'S pigment-spot treatment uses a blend of antioxidants and over forty different herbs and fruits. "Vitamin C, vitamin E, the citruses—where those vitamins come from. Grape seed extract, omega-3, omega-6 fatty acids—they're all antioxidants."

Wrinkles

SHELLEY notes that hydration is a big part of preventing wrinkles. So is wearing sunscreen every day. "Even when it's cloudy there are still UV rays." When clients come to her for help with wrinkles, she applies Elina's all-natural products and uses modern equipment. "I have a cold-laser machine, which exercises the muscles, and tones and lifts the skin."

Beyond that, there is aging gracefully. "You know what? We're going to wrinkle. It's not about completely preventing them. It's about taking care of ourselves. It goes with the whole well-balanced life: diets, supplements, exercise."

She notes that wrinkles on the upper chest and neck may come from spraying perfume there. "If you wear perfume, put it where the sun don't shine. The saleswomen selling these products probably don't even know that. The cosmetic and skin-care industry is very underregulated. They pretty much can say and claim anything. There are twenty thousand chemicals in cosmetic and skin-care products, and only a small percentage of them are tested by the FDA."

On Cosmetic Surgery

MARIANNE has many clients "who eat very healthily and do everything healthy—then they go shoot Botox into their system. When it comes to beauty they are prepared to take chances because they want to look good. I think the majority of women will do anything to look good. Everybody has their breasts done, their thighs, and their faces. There are medical aestheticians who do all these procedures, and medi-spas.

"There are two movements: There's the natural movement, and then there's the other movement. I think the other movement is getting stronger. I can see that by the fact that there are not that many pure products on the market. Most of them have some kind of harsh ingredients. Using organic products makes a difference too, but it may take a little time; results are not immediate or overnight.

"I don't want to do Botox; I don't want to put botulism in my system. Most women will do anything to look young. But I think it's also the men. We are so programmed through the media and movie stars. It's all about how everybody looks younger, and it's about the men we seek feedback from. But there are also men who *don't* want that in women, who actually *prefer* natural-looking women, who see aging gracefully as important. And *I* really see that as important. In Europe you don't see as much plastic as you see here. Women look beautiful at every age.

"I wouldn't *want* to look thirty, actually. I think it's losing sight of the gift of life and the beauty of the natural cycle. There is so much beauty at every different age. When I see what it's like to be in my fifties, I wouldn't want to be younger. But I don't *know* what I would do after sixty.

"I think what's important is to be more connected to yourself. Then you won't feel a need to do surgery. The connection is what gives you vivacity and zest for life."

ELINA is adamantly in favor of noninvasive methods. "In order to look their best, women do not have to endanger their health with surgery, toxic products, or harmful procedures. But most people are not aware of alternative opportunities. Big corporations continue promoting extreme makeovers and toxic injections as the only solution for fighting the effects of aging. I deeply believe that holistic beauty procedures and natural skin-care products can deliver dramatic and long-lasting results without any of the health risks associated with surgical face lifts and other cosmetic procedures."

Elina put this viewpoint to the test. "After seeing so many expensive and health-risking cosmetic surgeries performed on TV, we decided to produce our own makeover show. We demonstrated noninvasive and very effective techniques to rejuvenate the skin and spirit of five female volunteers, all over the age of fifty. Before coming to us, all of them were considering surgeries or Botox. After one month of facial treatments and Elina Skin Care product use, they completely changed their mind. They not only looked better (and younger!) physically, they felt much more confident in their daily lives." (For a DVD of the show, e-mail elina@elinaskincare.com.)

JOHN teaches his acupuncture patients a chi gung facial massage technique to reduce stress. "It helps increase the blood flow, which then increases the turnover of the epithelial tissues, and works to stimulate the muscles so that they actually start being reactivated and kind of pull the tissue up into place. It's really shocking how little has to be done to create a really major effect. And they can continue to do the techniques between treatments and for years after the treatments, and then they don't have to come see me as often." Inviting anyone to try it out, he suggests, "If you sit and look in the mirror and put your finger over one of the jaw muscles and move it a quarter of an inch, you might look ten years younger. By making just tiny movements adjusting the muscle, you'll see big differences as it pulls the skin back into place."

Regarding cosmetic surgery, he says, "I'm not a proponent of cosmetic surgery, but I'm not 100 percent against it, either. I know someone who had the lower part of her face done some years ago, and overall I think it was beneficial to her. She's a real estate broker in Pasadena, a job that's related to looking good. I think the surgery and the effects she got from it were probably more helpful than not. But I think that's in the minority. I think the negative things are there, including the negative possibilities that go along with surgery in general and all the psychological issues, such as people becoming addicted to the surgery.

"In Chinese medicine, we look at the meridians, the chi flow through the body. Frequently, depending on how deeply they go, those surgeries will cut the meridians, or at least scar them. Whenever you scar the body, you are disrupting the ability to get electromagnetic flow across that scar. That really does change things there. I worked with an acupuncturist years ago, and the first question she would ask was 'Do you have any scars?' And before she would do anything else, she would get the energy flowing around those scars, and it was just amazing what would happen to people."

KAREN has brought her more than fifteen years of research on selenium and vitamin E to address helping the skin recover from laser-abrasion procedures as well as other kinds of wound healing. On the subject of how selenium delivered topically as L-selenomethionine, coupled with vitamin E, can help the skin recover, she said, "They're both good antioxidants and both are known to be anti-inflammatory. It stood to reason that they would help in wound healing, too." Her latest study convinced her of the combined healing and inflammation-reduction properties of the two. The vitamin E needs to be in the form of d-alpha-tocopherol, with a minimum concentration of 2 to 5 percent for efficacy. The selenium needs to be in the form of L-selenomethionine, the only kind absorbed by the skin.

When to See a Dermatologist

MARIANNE advises seeing a dermatologist if any of the following apply:

- You have sun scabs on your face that don't want to heal.

- You see any unusual marks on the face.

- You have skin cancer in any way, because it's critical to catch it early. It's not necessarily dangerous to your health, but you could end up having a big chunk cut of out of your face and needing plastic surgery.

- You have acne to the degree that you just can't live with it.

- You have rosacea, depending on how bad it is. Rosacea is hard to cure, but seeing a dermatologist might help re-press it.

- A skin condition that doesn't improve or go away.

She adds, "I think everybody should see a dermatologist once a year for a face and body check, especially if they're fair-skinned, in order to check for sun damage. With the ozone layer thinning, we've all become more sensitive to sun damage."

SHELLEY notes that "dermatologists aren't educated on skin *care*; they're educated on skin *diseases*. If my clients have a big hormonal imbalance, I can provide a certain amount of care externally; but when there's an internal problem going on, sometimes I'll refer them to my acupuncturist [John Nieters] to work on it internally. Or I refer them if their skin is really red and inflamed and cystic, and I can tell it's not getting better."

ELINA declares firmly, "You *never* have to see a traditional dermatologist. If a child comes in to a dermatologist, they get started on antibiotics. Usually, children start to have acne because their hormones get imbalanced and they produce a little bit too much oil, and that oil plugs their pores and they start having simple acne at age thirteen or fourteen. Most teenagers have that. Unfortunately, most dermatologists *only* prescribe antibiotics. So it's the worst place to go for skin problems.

"People don't need antibiotics; they need a proper cleansing regimen and anti-inflammatory herbal products, which will help them reduce the bacterial activity in the skin. I don't mind if somebody has no other choice than to take antibiotics, but you need to try healthier ways first. People need to go to holistic skin-care specialists, where their pores will be deeply cleaned, where they will be trained how to take care of their skin and have the right topical products. I train holistic aestheticians—Shelley is one. I work with a whole network of M.D.s who work holistically. You can have alternatives. You're responsible for your health."

KAREN says, "If you have any disease of the skin, you should go to a dermatologist so we can help. Like if you have a rash, an allergy, or bad acne. The over-the-counter drugs are never as strong as the medicine a doctor can give, and the medicine a doctor can give is usually cheaper. And going to a doctor once or twice usually solves the situation."

ADDITIONAL ADVICE FROM OUR EXPERTS

Marianne Damhuis
The Importance of Pleasure

"Doing things that you enjoy is really good for you—dancing, love, deep spiritual connection, nature, harmony, balance. If you're so busy being so strict about everything that you don't have any pleasure, then that's not going to show through in your skin.

"Take time for yourself. Take a really nice hot/cold, hot/cold, hot/cold shower—you get out of that shower and you feel really good! You won't even feel like putting your clothes on. Or just wrap yourself in a sarong and sit down and do some really nice breathing. You will start to feel good about your whole self. Take an air bath when you can. If you have any privacy, just walk around naked for a while, just to feel the sun on you, just to feel the air on your body without clothes, just to be more touched and more aware. We are sensual, and these are all ways of connecting to the senses and our body. Go somewhere in nature and become aware of your connection to everything."

Digesting Your Life

"I think the biggest thing is to be able to get into your body and feel yourself. And to feel all your emotions, including anger or whatever it is. If you could just sit for a minute, feel where it is, and feel that feeling 100 percent, it kind of changes. You're not pushing it away or suppressing it or avoiding it; you're just integrating it, letting everything *be*. So you can glow and feel good because you're digesting and assimilating everything—your food, your emotions, *life*. I think just taking supplements and medication—it doesn't get assimilated in the body."

Beauty from Within

"I see beauty as life, and living life, digesting life. Everything is going to show on your face, in the skin. Some of this is genetic: Some people have better skin than others; some do next to nothing for their skin and they look great. So it's not that you can do one thing and you'll have beautiful skin. You just do the best you can with what you have. The beauty comes from within. And if it's not flawless skin, so what, if there's nothing else that goes with it?"

Balance

"What's important is to be comfortable in your own skin: to have water on it, and air on it, and eat well, and just feel good about yourself. And touch. It's about balance—not being addicted to drama, going up and down and finding ways to get stimulated. I think that shows up in the skin, too. I also think keeping your weight steady makes a difference. If you are seesawing all the time with your weight, you lose elasticity, so that shows on the skin, too."

Being in Touch with Yourself

"Feel the effects for yourself. Even with vitamins. And with the sun: You can feel when it's okay and when it's not. Pay attention. If we don't pay attention, we keep thinking, 'Here's the formula; I'll do that.' So it works for some and it doesn't work for others. Because we're all unique.

"If you start by doing things that you feel are good for you, you'll start to feel better about yourself. Even if you start in a small way, like by cutting out something that you feel is not good, you will start to feel the effects and will start to go more into a positive way of doing things. Sometimes you need a kick start. It takes a lot of discipline to stay balanced. So that's why if you just start with a little thing, even taking some vitamins, you start to feel better about yourself. And you start to feel motivated to take care of yourself.

"I find that when people who don't usually have facials do have one, they get motivated to take care of themselves. They relax very deeply, reach a place where they see another side of themselves a little bit, and decide they want to nurture how 'not to sweat the small stuff.' When you relax deeply in yourself, everything else can kind of fall away and you start to get more perspective on things and then to take some more time out simply for that."

Using Natural Cosmetic Products

Marianne is devoted to totally pure ingredients. "All the cosmetic companies come out with these ingredients that say 'vitamins,'" she declares, "but vitamins comprise such a small fraction of the ingredients and are therefore not going to do anything. They say 'natural ingredients,' but if you look at the ingredients, there are some things in there that aren't natural. They all need preservatives. It's all just hype."

Instead, she uses a brand called Eminence—"organic, very pure. As far as I can see, these products are the purest on the market. They actually check the ingredients, they're very careful, and they preserve their products through the fruit acids, salicylic acid." Unlike products that use a lot of salicylic acid, which thins the skin, "Eminence uses less than 1 percent, just to preserve the product. Most aestheticians use a lot of different things from different companies, but I don't use anything else." Eminence is only sold in spas and salons, or on the Internet (www.eminenceorganics.com).

On Touch

"Touch is an important part of well-being. Everybody needs to be touched. I can feel that a lot of my clients are not often touched, that their skin is hungry for that. Maybe they have sexual touch, but that's very different from loving touch or healing touch. Any loving touch is good. If you have no partner or you don't get good touch from a partner, you can get a massage or facial. When I give clients a facial or a massage, I see their faces change. They get 'wider,' and the lines decrease. Maybe it would be longer-lasting if they could stay in that space for a while. Healing touch keeps your mind on your body and on your skin." Having a healing facial brings people back to a more tender time "when you were little and had your face washed."

We often underrate the importance of our skin, especially facial skin. "The skin has all this memory. We hold so much in our face. And the face is really such a tender place. It's the first part of the body to take in impressions, or to defend us. There's just so much that goes on in the face."

Becoming Conscious

"It's important to give yourself attention and love, consciously. Knowing what you're putting on your face, appreciating the smells, the texture, everything. Not putting on a product absentmindedly but really *feeling* it in your face. Trace the lines in your face, pat your face—just totally be present with it, instead of just putting the product on and doing something else.

Even that small thing penetrates through your whole being. The senses are a way into the spirit. Spirit is your connection to yourself and nature and the whole thing."

Your Daily Beauty Routine

"It's important to have a daily beauty routine in the morning and at night. Most important is cleansing, exfoliating, and moisturizing. Exfoliate once a day or once a week, depending on the exfoliator. I do it in the shower. And cleanse your face twice a day. In the morning, exfoliate or cleanse, then use a moisturizer and a sunscreen. At night, the same thing: Use a moisturizer or, if your skin is quite dry, a good night cream. Toner is important too. And a masque—you can just get in the bathtub and put a nice masque on your face, sit back, and re-lax. It feels so good."

Shelley Rosenfeld

Shelley analyzes her clients' skin to determine "whether it's oily, dry, sensitive, has broken capillaries, rosacea, pigmenta-tion, and so on," and she targets each facial treatment toward the skin's needs, using herbs, minerals, and essential oils. "I make an herbal tea blend and put compresses on their face. Some tea blends calm the skin down; some get the circulation going. Each facial is different."

Skin Type vs. Skin Condition

Everyone has an inborn skin *type*, as well as a skin *condition*, based on personal and environmental stresses. "Stress can dry the skin out and cause breakouts. Even brown spots can be caused by trauma. Hormones, sun, and trauma all affect the condition of the skin. So I use products that are appropriate for the skin *type*, but I'm treating the *condition* of the skin.

"All people know if their skin is oily or dry. But there's a difference between being *dry* and being *dehydrated*. Being *dry* means that genetically they don't produce a lot of oil in their oil glands; being *dehydrated* means there's not enough water content. The skin is usually the first part of the body to show dehydration, because our inner organs need the hydration first. Dehydration is what makes the skin feel tight."

Cosmetic Products

"A lot of what's available via over-the-counter products deals with skin *type*—whether we're oily or dry—but it doesn't so much deal with *condition:* redness, dilated capillaries, brown spots. Over-the-counter acne medication actually dries out the skin. And the skin's oil and water content needs to be balanced. So I'm a big proponent of getting skin-care treatments. There are also natural things you can do at home.

"A lot of the ingredients of the products Elina makes that I use include sea buckthorn, amber, organic sulfur. I use liquid chlorophyll on the skin to calm it down; powdered goat's milk helps with the brown spots. Everything I use is natural. I learned it all from her. When we take vitamins internally, only 20 percent get to our skin, because our inner organs absorb and use them first. Using *topical* vitamins enables them to get to the skin. Elina's products are herbs; they're yellow and brown. Her products aren't white because there's no wax in them. The antioxidant helps heal the skin, and it helps with collagen production. As we get older our collagen, which gives the skin its plumpness, slows down in its production. To a certain extent, there are topical things that we can do to increase collagen levels.

"Most products just go to the *epi*dermis of the skin. Because their carriers are thick creams, they have big molecules, which don't get into the skin. Elina's products go to the *dermis*, where collagen and elastin are produced, so they get into the blood. The results I get using natural products are amazing. People's skin is more evenly toned, it's fresher looking, and acne is much improved. I'm not about fear—'Oh my gosh, you're aging!' And the clients who are attracted to me happen to be more natural, don't wear makeup, and are okay with aging gracefully."

Protect Yourself with Knowledge

Reading the labels is important. "Avoid products with mineral oil, petrolatum, parabens, sodium lauryl sulfate, alcohol, propylene glycol, artificial colors or fragrances, and phtalates. These ingredients are toxic. A lot of over-the-counter brands use formaldehyde to provide a long shelf life, so people are actually putting formaldehyde on their skin. Skin-care companies use them because they are inexpensive. Just because products are fancy doesn't mean they're good. It just means they spend a lot of money on marketing. You can look up any ingredients on the Internet to become more conscious and responsible about what you're putting on your skin: www.safecosmetics.org and www.ewg.org."

Daily Beauty Routine

1. Cleanse with a facial cleanser. Soap is bad for the skin—it has a really high pH so it strips the face of any oil, completely dehydrating the skin. For dry skin, milky cleansers are better; for oily skin, those that foam up are better.

2. Exfoliate to remove the dead skin cells. As we age, the production of enzymes that shed dead skin slows down. Exfoliants speed up the process. For thicker skin, every day is good; for thinner skin, twice a week.

3. Moisturize.

4. Protect with sunblock.

Elina Fedotova
Natural, Organic Skin-Care Products

Elina makes her own skin- and body-care products from all-natural, organic ingredients. Her product line changes with the season: "If you constantly eat the same soup, you get sick of it, and the same happens with skin-care products." Her ingredients include, among others, chamomile; burdock root; sea buckthorn; Baltic amber; proteins; vitamins such as C palmitate, D, and E; grape seed extract; wheat germ extract; kojic acid; and licorice root. The active ingredients are extracted naturally from plants and vegetables.

Delivering the Benefits Through the Skin

Elina makes a blend of herbal infusions that encapsulate lyposomes for deep delivery into the dermis. "We can't really deeply affect the skin without making very deeply penetrating, transdermal products. One way is to encapsulate all active ingredients into the lyposome. Lyposomes act like a vehicle delivering those anti-inflammatory superantioxidants—very healing ingredients—deep into the dermis." This contrasts with most skin-care products, which are emulsified by white, synthetic waxes. "Even if they contain beneficial herbs, those herbs never have a chance to penetrate through the skin barrier to the dermis."

She uses many of the herbs recommended in the FACE program. "Siberian ginseng energizes, restores, and repairs skin on a cellular level, for a more firming and youthful look. And grape seed extract is a powerful antioxidant for restoring the skin. When people start to take grape seed extract, very often they have fewer pigment spots, fewer liver spots, or fewer sun-damage spots.

"All my herbs include antioxidants. For example, in one jar of my antiwrinkle moisturizer, there is horsetail, ginseng, black currant (a very powerful antioxidant), gotu kola (also a very powerful antioxidant), chamomile, plantain, horse chestnut (a very powerful anti-inflammatory), and St. John's wort (a very powerful antidepressant and anti-inflammatory herb). They're all in my products. You can eat my products with a spoon and get calm and relaxed and reduce your cortisol level."

Aromatherapy Can Be Good for Your Skin

Stress can also be reduced by natural beautiful aromas, and all the products contain a blend of aromatherapeutic oils. "People like to use my antiwrinkle moisturizer in the morning, which has a blend of essential oils like ylang ylang, sandalwood, and lavender. Lavender is very relaxing and calming. Sandalwood and ylang ylang are very beneficial for skin and are also an aphrodisiac combination, so you feel more sensual, more relaxed, more happy. If you feel happy, you don't feel stressed. If you don't feel stressed, your cortisol levels go down."

The Importance of Reading the Label

Elina notes how rarely people read labels on cosmetic products, or understand the nature of the ingredients. "Skin-care products should provide *nourishment* for your skin, like food provides nourishment for your entire body. I don't have anything in my products that wouldn't be individually beneficial. Instead of using emulsifying waxes, I use soy salicylates. If the emulsion is made from toxic waxes or petroleum jelly or artificial things, it's as if you made a soup from organic vegetables and diluted them in a plastic bag. The whole solution should be beneficial, and there shouldn't be such a difference between active and nonactive ingredients."

She strongly recommends analyzing skin-care products before buying them, particularly by reading the label in search of good ingredients. "A company can mix a few ingredients and call that solution by a certain trade name. That's why it's so important to analyze the ingredients." She suggests doing a computer search on Google or Yahoo to get the definitions of the ingredients.

Put (Organic) Food on Your Face

"Instead of using questionable skin-care products that are full of preservatives and waxes, if you have good food in your refrigerator—organically grown vegetables and fruits, yogurt made from organic milk with active probiotics (e.g., by Horizon), and no highly processed foods—you can wash your face with yogurt or organic buttermilk. This will be much better than soapy cleansers full of detergents like sodium lauryl sulfate, which causes blindness in rats. And you can crush organic fruits and vegetables in the blender and make a mask. Mix it with organic oatmeal. Oatmeal has all sorts of nutrients for your skin." She also suggests using olive oil as a moisturizer, and a blend of papaya (papain) and pineapple (bromelain) as an exfoliator.

"If I lost my products or suitcase while traveling, I would never go and buy commercial products. I would go to a health food store and buy some food. I would put on avocado to soften my face: I would use cucumbers on my eyes. Most of the foods are very good masks. You can survive for a while only using foods." Food can supplement your skin's health, too. "It won't hurt to crush some fruits and vegetables several times a week and apply them to your face as a mask for extra effect; for instance, try organic strawberries. I'm stressing *organic* because it means it's been grown without toxic fertilizers, herbicides, and pesticides. If you have that good food and are eating well and are applying those masks, you probably won't have any stress. You'll enjoy your aromatherapy time, eat well, put good food on your face, and, of course, if you use my products, your skin will be looking young."

Your Daily Beauty Routine

"There are three basic steps: cleanse, tone, and moisturize. Cleanse with a cleanser specially formulated for your face. Don't use soap!" The products and regimen to use depend upon your skin type—dry to normal; normal to oily; sun-damaged; acne-prone. The following are Elina's basic steps for caring for the two most common types:

Dry to normal skin

In the morning

1. Moisten face and apply Elina's Gentle Cleanser and Eye Makeup Remover. Lather gently with circular motions. Rinse well. Pat dry.

2. Mist face with Botanical Toner for Dry and Sensitive Skin. Pat dry with tissue or cotton.

3. Smooth a small amount of Elite Formula over face.

4. Apply Intensive Eye Revitalization Complex around eye and/or neck area as needed.

5. Use Ambra Lift to lift, revitalize, and energize skin.

6. Moisturize with Elina Sun Shelter Makeup.

In the evening

1. Use Gentle Cleanser and Eye Makeup Remover, as in the morning.

2. Use Botanical Toner for Dry and Sensitive Skin, as in the morning.

3. Smooth a small amount of Cream for Dry and Mature Skin over face.

4. Apply Intensive Eye Revitalization Complex, as in the morning.

Normal to oily skin

In the morning

1. Moisten face and apply Gentle Cleanser for Oily Skin. Lather gently with circular motions. Rinse well. Pat dry.

2. Mist face with Alcohol-Free Herbal Toner. Pat dry with tissue or cotton.

3. Apply Oil Control Formula over oily or acne-prone areas to minimize pores and eliminate bacteria.

4. Smooth a small amount of Anti-Wrinkle Liposome Moisturizer over dry areas of face.

5. Apply Intensive Eye Revitalization Complex around eye and/or neck area as needed.

6. Use Ambra Lift to lift, revitalize, and energize skin.

7. Apply Oil-Free Mineral Makeup.

In the evening

1. Use Gentle Cleanser and Eye Makeup Remover, as in the morning.

2. Use Alcohol-Free Herbal Toner, as in the morning.

3. Smooth a small amount of Super Antioxidant Liposome Night Cream over face.

4. Apply Intensive Eye Revitalization Complex around eye and/or neck area as needed.

John Nieters
Acupuncture Rebalances the Nervous System

Acupuncture is a Chinese system that is at least six thousand years old in which tiny needles are inserted at key points into the body, along energy pathways called meridians. When the body is functioning at full health capacity, energy (chi) flows freely through the meridians. When there is illness, disease, or malfunction of any kind, the energy does not flow freely. Acupuncture can redress this situation by rebalancing the sympathetic and parasympathetic nervous systems.

Stress and the Skin

"It's a little different from Western medicine," John states. For example, "In Chinese medicine we would talk about a health situation in many terms—say, 'coursing the liver and rectifying the chi.' That means changing the blood flow, allowing a different level of energetic movement. Physiologically, it lowers your sympathetic nervous system response. It changes your neurotransmitter patterns, your hormone patterns, so that you can actually go into a more profound level of relaxation. *Because when you're in a high sympathetic nervous system state, in a high adrenal-function state such as would occur when facing a tiger, healing is a very low priority.* And the stress hormones that are released are extremely damaging to the skin. They are *catabolic*—they *destroy* tissue—rather than being *anabolic*, which *builds* tissue. So whenever you're under stress, it wears out *all* of your tissues. And one of the places that shows up the most is on the skin.

"When you undergo acupuncture, it will *downgrade* the sympathetic nervous system and *upgrade* the parasympathetic so your body can heal. With the skin, this becomes critical, because as we age the turnover rate of tissue becomes much slower. So when we're younger, turnover might be every twenty to thirty days; by the time you're in your fifties, it might be every sixty days. So the skin, physically, is just a lot older. And if it's being broken down by external problems or by a lack of internal nourishment, it just wears out horribly.

"So I work with patients to rebalance that stress reaction. I teach all of my cosmetic acupuncture patients some breathing techniques, or some way of creating relaxation. Because this makes a huge difference in the success of the treatment."

There are three major ways to go when it comes to treatment with acupuncture:

1. **Increase the chi in the blood:** "This works by *stimulating*—primarily in acupuncture points. We use a lot of very tiny needles on the face, perhaps sixty or seventy. We do what we call an 'apex technique,' where we use three needles in very close proximity. This means we don't have to needle as deeply or use as large a needle, and we still get a great effect. It does what acupuncture is designed to do—increase blood flow and 'chi flow' to

the area. People will get very tingly; their faces will feel
like they're coming alive again."

2. **Create a collagen matrix:** "We will do 'threading techniques'—using longer needles, and placing needles under the skin, especially in deep furrows and areas where
the tissue is really broken down, and where the collagen
matrix has been pretty much destroyed. This causes the
body to sense that it's been attacked, and it starts to
bring more collagen to the site, causing a kind of a micro-
scarring underneath the surface, which will plump up or
fill out the tissue. It's like getting a collagen injection,
except it's your *own* collagen. That's a really good technique in people with very deep lines on or near the forehead or along the nasal/labial groove below the nose."

3. **Reactivate the macrophage system:** "When you needle
into any particular site on the body, whether it's an
acupuncture point or not, it draws the body's attention
to that area. There's now a Western technique called
prolotherapy. It's becoming very popular for treatment of
disk and athletic injuries. The therapist puts in a hypo-
dermic needle and injects some substance that will irri-
tate the area. Then the body says, 'Oh, wait a minute,
there's an injury here. We better go back and fix it.' So
the macrophages—the huge cells that come and eat debris in the body—get reactivated and come back to that
injury site. At a certain point in the injury process, the
body seems to kind of forget about it, and frequently the
injury will not heal completely. But if you then go back
and do acupuncture into that site, the body will go back
and do more healing."

Finding a Facial Acupuncturist in Your Area

"It's easier to find people now who actually have been trained
to do facial acupuncture, specifically. Cosmetic acupuncture

sites are now available on the Internet. If you Google it, a couple of major schools will show up, and they recommend practitioners."

CONCLUDING WORDS…

A few last pieces of advice from our experts:

MARIANNE DAMHUIS "The body is always moving toward healing itself. So what you want to do is give it the optimum environment to heal itself."

SHELLEY ROSENFELD "Taking care of the skin shouldn't be an obsession. It should just be part of eating well and taking a holistic approach to life."

ELINA FEDATOVA "When you want to look amazing for a special occasion, you most likely head to your favorite store. Or maybe you will come to the conclusion that the dress that will make you look the best should be designed specifically for you. But how many times will you wear this dress that you went to great lengths for? Probably just once or twice. However, you wear your skin for life."

JOHN NIETERS "I see that people get such good results when they do a nutritional program and see someone like Shelley for facials and then do the chi gung work in facial acupuncture. The feedback is just fabulous."

KAREN BURKE "Larry Dossey, M.D., wrote a book called *The Body Is the Healer,* and I agree. The body regulates itself. We don't necessarily need more of everything all the time."

… AND MY OWN CONCLUDING THOUGHTS

Committing yourself to a beauty regime of reducing stress through the FACE program and following the pathways of natural skin care suggested here will gradually show you a difference in what your life can be. Beauty really is an inside job, and you now have all the tools to do it. Over time, a truly beautiful face will be yours, and you'll know it from the inside out as well as the outside in.

. . . .
. .
.

Recipes

Here is an entire week of delicious breakfast, lunch, and dinner recipes—seven recipes for each meal. Feel free to mix and match them each day according to your tastes. And when you can't treat yourself to one of these outstanding meals, keep the Helping Hand "rules" in mind and combine your carbs, fats, and proteins accordingly.

These recipes have been specially crafted for us by New York City chef Michael Saccone. Each meal has been created to incorporate as many FACE-friendly nutrients as possible. Since age fourteen, Michael Saccone has worked for many restaurants, catering companies, and clubs. Most notably, he apprenticed at George Perrier's Le Bec Fin in Philadelphia, worked at the four-star Le Cirque in New York City, and cooked privately for several high-profile clients. As a private chef, he has gained experience in health-conscious cooking. Currently he is employed by Maury Povich at his television studio and in his family home. Michael is also the owner of City Chef Corporation, which produces prepared side dishes that accompany meats, poultry, and seafood for Manhattan's top specialty markets. Michael resides in New York City with his wife, Adrienne, and two young children, Catherine and Elizabeth.

Bon appétit!

BREAKFAST

. . . .

Oatmeal Blueberry Pancakes with Almond Butter

PER SERVING: 502 CALORIES (KCAL) ~ 28 G FAT ~ 11 G SATURATED FAT
177 MG CHOLESTEROL ~ 14 G PROTEIN ~ 827 MG SODIUM
49 G CARBOHYDRATE ~ 6 G FIBER ~ 20 G SUGAR ~ 366 MG CALCIUM

*Pancakes made with oats, some flour, buttermilk,
and dense with blueberries, topped with butter
creamed with sweetened almond paste*

½ cup all-purpose flour
1 cup rolled oats
½ tablespoon baking powder
½ tablespoon baking soda
½ teaspoon salt
1½ cups buttermilk or milk
2 tablespoons peanut oil
3 eggs, separated
1 pint blueberries
½ stick soft butter (plus extra for cooking—about 1 tablespoon)
2 ounces almond paste or marzipan

Grind the almond paste and butter in a bowl with the back of
a spoon or in a food processor until well incorporated and
smooth. Set aside.

Sift together dry ingredients. In a large bowl, beat yolks
and gradually add peanut oil and then buttermilk. Beat egg
whites to soft peaks.

Start to heat grill pan or skillet over medium heat.

Gradually stir dry ingredients into yolk mixture, stopping
when ingredients are just combined. Fold in beaten whites,
starting with a little to lighten the mixture and then adding
the rest. Fold in blueberries.

Test skillet with a drop of water (it should sizzle, not instantly evaporate). Add about a teaspoon of butter to pan, swirling it to coat entire surface. When butter is sizzling but not yet brown, ladle out pancakes. The pancakes should look firm and have well-formed dimples when you flip them. Brown flipped side and cook next batch, adding butter as necessary. Serve hot with almond butter spread over the cakes, like on toast.

Serves 4.

·   ·   ·   ·   ·

Smoked Salmon and Arugula Omelet

PER SERVING: 298 CALORIES (KCAL) ~ 19 G FAT ~ 5 G SATURATED FAT
437 MG CHOLESTEROL ~ 24 G PROTEIN ~ 1,929 MG SODIUM
6 G CARBOHYDRATE ~ 1 G FIBER ~ 3 G SUGAR ~ 102 MG CALCIUM

Omelet stuffed with smoked salmon and peppery arugula and sautéed with Bermuda onion

1 tablespoon olive oil
1 small Bermuda onion
1 bunch arugula
½ tablespoon capers
1 pinch red pepper flakes
4 large eggs
1 tablespoon milk
½ teaspoon salt
4 ounces smoked salmon

Skin onion, remove core, cut in half, and slice into ⅛-inch slices.

Place sauté pan over medium heat, add about ½ tablespoon of olive oil and onions, and cook onions until soft, flipping occasionally—about four minutes.

Trim stems from arugula, wash in large bowl with cold water, remove leaves, and shake off water.

Turn up heat on onions, add a little more olive oil if necessary, the red pepper flakes, capers, and arugula, along with a pinch of salt. Cook greens, tossing frequently, until greens wilt, about a minute. Place mixture in a strainer that is resting in a bowl. Wipe pan with a paper towel and return to stovetop, reducing heat to medium.

Scramble eggs with milk and salt. Add about another ½ tablespoon of olive oil to pan and swirl around. When a test drop of water sputters, add eggs to pan. Let the eggs start to set for a few seconds, and stir gently with a spatula, allowing eggs to set a little again before continuing to stir. When eggs are about two-thirds cooked, reduce heat to low and allow omelet to take shape. Place greens mixture along the center, from twelve to six o'clock, and top with salmon. When eggs are done, flip one side over to shape omelet, and then slide omelet onto serving dish.

Makes one large omelet that serves 2.

＊　　＊　　＊　　＊　　＊

Sweet Breakfast Biscuits and Gingered Prunes

PER SERVING: 454 CALORIES (KCAL) ~ 13 G FAT ~ 7 G SATURATED FAT
77 MG CHOLESTEROL ~ 7 G PROTEIN ~ 281 MG SODIUM
78 G CARBOHYDRATE ~ 5 G FIBER ~ 33 G SUGAR ~ 204 MG CALCIUM

*Breakfast "cookies" made with toasted millet and
served with stewed gingered prunes*

¼ cup hulled millet seeds
⅔ cup water
1 cup all-purpose flour
2 teaspoons baking powder
⅓ cup sugar
4 tablespoons butter
1 egg
1 teaspoon vanilla
1 one-inch piece fresh ginger, peeled
1 cup pitted prunes

Toast millet in saucepan over medium-low heat until golden and starting to pop. Add water, cover pan, and reduce heat to low; cook until liquid is gone, about fifteen minutes.

Cream butter and sugar; add egg and vanilla. Sift together flour and baking powder into butter mixture. Stir in toasted millet.

Place spoonfuls of mixture on sheet pan lightly coated with nonstick spray or parchment paper. Bake for about twelve minutes or until golden. Let cool on sheet.

Slice ginger in half and add to small saucepan with prunes. Add just enough water to cover; bring to a gentle simmer. Cook for twenty minutes, transfer to a bowl, and refrigerate until cool and a thick syrup has formed, about three hours.

Yields eight biscuits; serves 4.

*   *   *   *   *

Crunchy Yogurt Parfait

PER SERVING: 369 CALORIES (KCAL) ~ 5 G FAT ~ 0 G SATURATED FAT
0 MG CHOLESTEROL ~ 7 G PROTEIN ~ 141 MG SODIUM
76 G CARBOHYDRATE ~ 9 G FIBER ~ 47 G SUGAR ~ 142 MG CALCIUM

*Parfait made with alternating layers of berries,
vanilla yogurt, and granola*

½ pint blueberries
½ pint raspberries
2 tablespoons honey
2 granola bars, crumbled
1 cup low-fat vanilla yogurt

Place berries into separate bowls; stir 1 tablespoon of honey into each bowl, coating berries well. Place in refrigerator for one hour, gently stirring every fifteen minutes.

In two parfait cups or tall glasses, spoon alternating layers as follows: yogurt, granola, blueberries, yogurt, granola, raspberries, yogurt, and a final sprinkle of granola.

Serves 2.

Buckwheat Hazelnut Muffins

PER SERVING: 349 CALORIES (KCAL) ~ 20 G FAT ~ 6 G SATURATED FAT
50 MG CHOLESTEROL ~ 7 G PROTEIN ~ 303 MG SODIUM
34 G CARBOHYDRATE ~ 4 G FIBER ~ 16 G SUGAR ~ 66 MG CALCIUM

*One of my personal breakfast favorites, these muffins
are made with buckwheat flour and are flavored
with hazelnut, orange, and raisins*

¾ cup raisins
1 orange
1 cup blanched hazelnuts, chopped
1¼ cups all-purpose flour
1 cup buckwheat flour
1 tablespoon baking powder
½ tablespoon baking soda
1 teaspoon salt
¼ teaspoon ground cloves
6 tablespoons butter
½ cup sugar
2 eggs
½ cup sour cream

Preheat oven to 375° F.

In a microwave-safe bowl, zest and juice orange. Add raisins. Cover with plastic and microwave for thirty seconds. Let sit to allow raisins to plump.

Toast hazelnuts on a sheet pan in oven.

Sift dry ingredients together.

Cream butter and sugar until fluffy. Continue mixing, adding one egg at a time, letting first egg fully incorporate before adding the second. Add sour cream and raisin mixture. Stir in dry ingredients until just uniformly mixed. Fold in hazelnuts.

Fill paper-lined muffin tin to ¾-height for each muffin. Bake about fifteen minutes or until golden. Let cool in pan.

Makes about 12 muffins.

Parmesan Florentine Eggs

PER SERVING: 391 CALORIES (KCAL) ~ 20 G FAT ~ 4 G SATURATED FAT
373 MG CHOLESTEROL ~ 24 G PROTEIN ~ 1,149 MG SODIUM
32 G CARBOHYDRATE ~ 10 G FIBER ~ 6 G SUGAR ~ 429 MG CALCIUM

Whole-grain toast topped with sautéed spinach, red peppers,
sliced olives, and finished with gratinéed eggs

2 bunches leaf spinach
1 sweet red pepper
¼ cup pitted Alfonzo olives
1 small shallot
½ tablespoon olive oil
4 eggs
1 teaspoon vinegar
3 ounces parmesan cheese, grated
2 slices seven-grain bread

Trim stems from spinach and place in large bowl filled with cold water. Lift leaves out and place in colander. Drain water, rinse bowl of sand, and repeat.

Cut pepper in half. Remove stem, seeds, and ribs and slice halves into ⅛-inch pieces.

Drain olives and cut into quarters. Peel shallot and mince.

Fill shallow pan with water and bring to a simmer. Add vinegar and crack eggs one at a time, gently releasing each egg into the water as close to the surface as possible. Poach the eggs to desired doneness.

While eggs poach, heat sauté pan over high heat, add about ½ tablespoon of olive oil, and add peppers. Sauté until soft; add shallot and cook another thirty seconds, tossing continuously. Add spinach and toss until wilted. Season with salt and pepper. Transfer to a strainer resting in a bowl, and allow to drain.

Toast bread on sheet pan under broiler, flipping to toast both sides. Place half the spinach mixture on each slice, making sure to cover bread completely. Next place two poached eggs on top of each bed of spinach mixture. Sprinkle with cheese and slide pan under the broiler again until cheese browns, about thirty seconds.

Serves 2.

*   *   *   *   *

Garden Frittata

PER SERVING: 232 CALORIES (KCAL) ~ 10 G FAT ~ 3 G SATURATED FAT
372 MG CHOLESTEROL ~ 15 G PROTEIN ~ 266 MG SODIUM
20 G CARBOHYDRATE ~ 2 G FIBER ~ 3 G SUGAR ~ 82 MG CALCIUM

Frittata crowded with broccoli, tomato, chard, and red onion, and bound with a bit of whole-wheat pasta

8 large eggs
2 ounces dry soba noodles
1 cup broccoli florets
1 bunch Swiss chard, trimmed and washed
1 tomato
1 yellow pepper
1 red onion
1 clove garlic, minced
1/8 teaspoon red pepper flakes
Salt to taste
1/2 tablespoon olive oil

Preheat oven to 350° F.

Bring a medium-sized pot of water to a boil. Add enough salt so that it tastes almost like the ocean. Fill a large bowl with ice water.

Cook broccoli in boiling salted water until tender, about two to three minutes. Pull out of water with a slotted spoon or spider, and plunge directly into ice water. Repeat with Swiss chard. Drain and set aside. Cook soba noodles in salt water and drain; set aside.

Remove stem end from tomato and cut in half east-west. With fingers, poke out the seeds while giving the tomato half a light squeeze. Chop tomato into ½-inch pieces.

Cut pepper in half; remove stem, seeds, and ribs. Slice into ⅛-inch slices.

Cut onion in half, remove the skin and the stem end, and slice into ⅛-inch slices.

Lightly beat the eggs.

Heat ovenproof nine-inch sauté pan (nonstick works best) over medium heat. Add about ½ tablespoon olive oil plus the onions. Sauté about three minutes and add peppers. When peppers are soft, add garlic and cook another thirty seconds; then add tomato, broccoli, Swiss chard, and soba noodles. Season aggressively with salt, and stir in beaten eggs. Turn heat to low and let cook about two minutes. Slide pan into oven and bake until set, about thirty minutes.

When done, slide frittata out of pan onto a serving platter. Cut into quarters and serve.

Serves 4.

LUNCH

· · · · · · · · · ·

Curry Chicken Salad

PER SERVING: 484 CALORIES (KCAL) ~ 23 G FAT ~ 4 G SATURATED FAT
30 MG CHOLESTEROL ~ 16 G PROTEIN ~ 169 MG SODIUM
60 G CARBOHYDRATE ~ 13 G FIBER ~ 41 G SUGAR ~ 211 MG CALCIUM

*Tender Boston lettuce and curried chicken sweetened
with green apples, raisins, and walnuts*

2 pounds chicken thighs
½ onion, chopped into fourths
1 celery stalk, chopped into fourths
1 carrot, chopped into fourths
1 bay leaf
4 green apples
¾ cup golden raisins
½ cup walnuts
2 heads Boston lettuce
½ cup low-fat plain yogurt
¼ cup mayonnaise
1 tablespoon curry powder
Salt and pepper to taste

Remove skin from chicken thighs, place into a medium
saucepan, fill with water until meat is covered by two inches.
Place pan over medium-high heat and bring to a gentle simmer. Skim off all the scum and fat that comes to the surface,
and add onion, celery, carrot, and bay leaf. Simmer for forty-
five minutes, skimming from time to time. Turn off heat and
transfer to a bowl; allow chicken to cool in broth.

Remove meat from thigh bones in large pieces; make
sure to remove vein. Dice meat into ½-inch cubes. Strain
broth and freeze for future use.

Dice two of the apples in ¼-inch cubes, leaving skin on.
Mix with walnuts and raisins.

Whisk together yogurt, mayonnaise, and curry powder until smooth. Fold in apple-nut mixture. Fold in chicken, and add salt and pepper to taste. Let sit, covered, in refrigerator.

Remove tough leaves and core from lettuce, and wash leaves in a large bowl of cold water. Spin dry. Arrange beds of lettuce on four plates. Slice remaining two green apples in half, remove core, and slice halves into ¼-inch slices. Arrange slices on lettuce, and distribute chicken salad in a mound over the apple slices and lettuce.

Serves 4.

＊　　＊　　＊　　＊　　＊

Gazpacho with Avocado Cream

PER SERVING: 299 CALORIES (KCAL) ~ 17G FAT ~ 2 G SATURATED FAT
0 MG CHOLESTEROL ~ 7 G PROTEIN ~ 764 MG SODIUM
34 G CARBOHYDRATE ~ 13 G FIBER ~ 16 G SUGAR ~ 124 MG CALCIUM

*Cold vegetable soup thick with celery, cucumber, sweet and
hot peppers, scallions, carrots, and tomato, flavored with
extra-virgin olive oil, red-wine vinegar, and herbs.
Serve with a hearty grain bread*

1 cucumber
1 carrot
2 ribs celery
1 tomato
1 green pepper
1 jalapeno pepper
4 scallions
⅛ cup chopped parsley
1 8-ounce can V8 juice
1 8-ounce can tomato juice
1 teaspoon Worcestershire sauce
1½ tablespoons red-wine vinegar
1 dash hot sauce
Salt and freshly ground black pepper
1 ripe avocado
½ lime

Salt and freshly ground black pepper
1 tablespoon extra-virgin olive oil

Peel carrot and cucumber. Remove seeds from cucumber by cutting lengthwise and scooping out with a spoon. Cut tomato in half east-west, and remove seeds and stem/core at top. Cut peppers in half and remove seeds, stems, and ribs. Fine-dice peppers and cucumber and set aside in large bowl.

Rough chop carrot, scallion, and celery. Pulse in food processor until finely chopped but not starting to lose liquid, and add to bowl. Repeat with tomato. Add parsley to bowl, as well as juices, Worcestershire, vinegar, and hot sauce. Adjust seasoning with salt and pepper. Chill well.

Cut avocado in half, remove pit, and scoop avocado meat from skin into processor. Add juice of ½ lime and process until smooth. Add salt and pepper to taste.

Ladle soup into chilled bowls and place a dollop of avocado in center. Lace top with a quick swirl of olive oil. Serve with hearty bread.

Serves 2.

* * * * *

Turkey Tabbouleh

PER SERVING: 492 CALORIES (KCAL) ~ 28 G FAT ~ 4 G SATURATED FAT
81 MG CHOLESTEROL ~ 28 G PROTEIN ~ 704 MG SODIUM
36 G CARBOHYDRATE ~ 8 G FIBER ~ 3 G SUGAR ~ 42 MG CALCIUM

Bulgur grain mixed with diced turkey breast, tomatoes, olives, scallion, and chopped parsley, finished with lemon and olive oil. Serve on a bed of shredded iceberg lettuce

1 cup bulgur grain
1 cup boiling water
1 teaspoon salt
2 tomatoes
½ cup pitted kalamata olives
1 bunch scallions

2 bunches flat-leaf parsley
1 large lemon
¼ cup olive oil
Salt and pepper
1 pound roast turkey breast
1 small head iceberg lettuce, shredded

Place bulgur and salt in a medium bowl; add boiling water, and cover with plastic wrap. Let soak until liquid is absorbed, about thirty-five minutes.

Cut tomatoes in half east-west, remove stem/core at top, and dice into ¼-inch pieces. Place into medium bowl and set aside. Trim and clean scallion in cold water and chop; add to tomatoes. Wash parsley in large bowl of cold water, shake or spin dry, and chop, avoiding stems. Slice olives and add to tomatoes with parsley. Dice turkey into ½-inch cubes and add to vegetables.

Remove plastic from bowl of bulgur, and fluff the grain with a fork. Juice the lemon and add to bulgur, along with olive oil, continuing to fluff with a fork. Add vegetables and turkey by fluffing in as well, and add salt and freshly ground pepper to taste.

Place lettuce on four plates and spoon tabbouleh over lettuce.

Serves 4.

·   ·   ·   ·   ·

Classic Club Broccoli Salad

PER SERVING: 369 CALORIES (KCAL) ~ 30 G FAT ~ 4 G SATURATED FAT
13 MG CHOLESTEROL ~ 14 G PROTEIN ~ 311 MG SODIUM
16 G CARBOHYDRATE ~ 8 G FIBER ~ 5 G SUGAR ~ 150 MG CALCIUM

*Crisp blanched broccoli tossed with bacon,
currants, and smoked almonds*

1 head broccoli
Salt

4 slices bacon
4 ounces smoked almonds (chopped, sliced, or whole)
¼ cup currants
⅓ cup mayonnaise
1 tablespoon distilled vinegar
1 tablespoon sugar
Salt and freshly ground black pepper

Fill a large bowl with ice water; set aside. Cut broccoli florets off the head in bite-size pieces. Bring a medium pot of water to a boil and add salt until it tastes almost like the ocean. Drop broccoli into boiling water and cook for one minute. Lift out broccoli with slotted spoon and plunge into bowl of ice water. When broccoli is cool, drain and place into colander to dry out.

Cook bacon in skillet or microwave until crisp. Crumble bacon, and mix in a bowl, along with smoked almonds and currants.

Whisk mayonnaise, vinegar, and sugar together. Fold in broccoli and nut mixture. Add salt and freshly ground pepper to taste.

Serves 4.

· · · · ·

Asian Shrimp Salad

PER SERVING: 250 CALORIES (KCAL) ~ 8 G FAT ~ 1 G SATURATED FAT
172 MG CHOLESTEROL ~ 27 G PROTEIN ~ 190 MG SODIUM
18 G CARBOHYDRATE ~ 3 G FIBER ~ 11 G SUGAR ~ 111 MG CALCIUM

Shrimp, sweet peppers, scallions, grapes, cilantro, and crushed peanuts dressed with a sweet-and-sour sauce

1 pound peeled raw shrimp
1 teaspoon Chinese five-spice powder
1 teaspoon salt
½ tablespoon peanut oil
1 red pepper
1 bunch scallions

1 carrot
1 bunch watercress
⅛ cup chopped cilantro
Juice of 1 lime
1 teaspoon fish sauce
1 tablespoon rice vinegar
1 teaspoon sugar
½ pound seedless grapes
¼ cup peanuts, crushed

Heat skillet over medium-high heat and test with water drop for fast sputter. Add peanut oil. Sprinkle shrimp with five-spice powder and salt, and sear in skillet on each side until firm and cooked (times vary based on size of shrimp, but about ninety seconds on each side should do). Set aside cooked shrimp to cool.

Wash scallions, and slice thinly on the diagonal into one-inch lengths. Core, seed, and remove ribs from pepper, and slice thinly into one-inch lengths. Trim ends from watercress, chop into one-inch lengths, wash in cold water, and spin dry. Combine all vegetables in a large bowl.

Whisk together lime juice, fish sauce, vinegar, and sugar. Pour over vegetables and toss. Place mixture on platter, arrange shrimp on top, and sprinkle with crushed peanuts. Garnish with grapes.

Serves 4.

*   *   *   *   *

Greek Luncheon Salad

PER SERVING: 530 CALORIES (KCAL) ~ 42 G FAT ~ 9 G SATURATED FAT
67 MG CHOLESTEROL ~ 22 G PROTEIN ~ 1,080 MG SODIUM
19 G CARBOHYDRATE ~ 6 G FIBER ~ 7 G SUGAR ~ 270 MG CALCIUM

Romaine and spinach garnished with cucumbers, tomato, olive, onion, and feta cheese. Topped with marinated chicken breast brushed with an herb vinaigrette

Two full boneless, skinless chicken breasts,
divided into halves, approximately 4 ounces each
2 lemons
½ cup olive oil
1 teaspoon dried oregano
1 small clove garlic, minced
¼ teaspoon freshly ground pepper
1 teaspoon salt
1 head romaine lettuce
1 bunch leaf spinach
1 cucumber
2 tomatoes
½ red onion
½ cup kalamata olives
8 ounces feta cheese

With the fine side of a box grater, grate the yellow part of the skin of one lemon. Place in jar or plastic container with lid. Add juice from both lemons, oregano, salt, pepper, garlic, and olive oil. Shake.

Place each halved chicken breast between plastic wrap and pound evenly until meat is about ½ inch thick all over. Place pieces in a broiler-safe pan, arranged so that they do not overlap. Pour a third of the dressing over them and turn to coat. Cover with plastic and place in refrigerator.

Trim and clean lettuce and spinach in a bowl of cold water. Lift leaves out and repeat washing with fresh cold water. Chop leaves into ¾-inch pieces and spin dry.

Cut cucumber in half lengthwise. Peel and seed cucumber, and slice halves into ¼-inch slices. Remove top stem/core of tomatoes and cut each into eight wedges. Slice onion half as thinly as possible.

Pat chicken dry with paper towel. Season with salt and pepper, and rub on some olive oil. Place into a pan under the oven broiler and cook through, flipping the breasts when halfway done. Remove from oven and brush breasts with some of the vinaigrette.

Toss leaves with remaining vinaigrette and adjust salt and ground pepper. Create a bed of leaves on each plate, arrange four tomato wedges on each, and equally distribute the cucumber, onion, olives, and feta cheese. Top each with a piece of chicken breast.

Serves 4.

. . . . .

Tuna Niçoise Salad

PER SERVING: 474 CALORIES (KCAL) ~ 23 G FAT ~ 3 G SATURATED FAT
100 MG CHOLESTEROL ~ 23 G PROTEIN ~ 536 MG SODIUM
47 G CARBOHYDRATE ~ 12 G FIBER ~ 7 G SUGAR ~ 156 MG CALCIUM

Green beans, tomato, hard-boiled egg, Niçoise olives, potatoes, and tuna on Bibb lettuce with a Dijon vinaigrette

2 eggs
1 tomato
4 ounces French green beans*
2 ounces Niçoise olives
¼ red onion
4 small red or yellow potatoes
1 teaspoon salt
1 6-ounce can tuna packed in olive oil
2 heads Bibb lettuce
1 teaspoon Dijon mustard
½ clove garlic, minced
Juice of one lemon
1 teaspoon sugar
¼ cup olive oil
1 pinch dried thyme

* French-style green beans, or *haricots verts*, are very thin. If they are unavailable, use regular green beans and slice them in half lengthwise.

Place eggs into a small pan, cover with water, and bring to a simmer over medium-high heat. Cover and turn off heat. After seven minutes remove eggs and plunge into ice water.

Place potatoes into small pan with water to cover and add salt. Bring to a simmer over medium-high heat, and cook until knife can easily penetrate. Cool.

Bring a medium-sized pan of water to a boil with enough salt to make it taste almost like the ocean. Trim beans and cook for two minutes. Remove with slotted spoon and plunge into ice water. When beans are cool, drain them.

Prepare vinaigrette by combining mustard, sugar, thyme, and garlic in a small bowl with a whisk. Add olive oil, a drop at a time at first to whisk into an emulsion. Gradually add remaining oil in a steady, thin stream while continuously whisking. Season with salt and fresh ground pepper.

Trim and wash lettuce and spin dry. Peel eggs and cut in quarters. Cut potatoes in quarters. Slice onion as thinly as possible. Core and cut tomato into wedges. Place lettuce on a platter, and arrange vegetables and eggs around perimeter. Place drained tuna in center, and garnish with olives. Serve vinaigrette on the side.

Serves 4.

DINNER

. . . .

Soba Primavera

PER SERVING: 649 CALORIES (KCAL) ~ 34 G FAT ~ 8 G SATURATED FAT
37 MG CHOLESTEROL ~ 29 G PROTEIN ~ 2,332 MG SODIUM
61 G CARBOHYDRATE ~ 2 G FIBER ~ 2 G SUGAR ~ 573 MG CALCIUM

*Japanese buckwheat noodles tossed with sautéed greens,
garlic, grape tomatoes, and olives, and topped
with parmesan cheese and chives*

2 bundles (about 4 ounces) soba noodles
1 tablespoon salt
1½ tablespoons olive oil
1 bunch kale, trimmed and washed
1 portobello mushroom, wiped clean and diced
½ cup grape tomatoes, halved
½ cup olives, sliced
1 clove minced garlic
1 shallot, peeled and thinly sliced
3 ounces parmesan, grated
⅓ bunch chives, chopped

Bring a medium-sized pot of salted water to a boil. Add soba
noodles and cook according to directions on package. Reserve
one cup of cooking water; drain noodles.

Heat large sauté pan over medium-high heat; add about
1 tablespoon of olive oil and the diced mushroom. Allow to
cook until released liquid has dried; add garlic, shallot, olives,
and tomato. Season with salt and pepper and cook another
two minutes. Put vegetables in a bowl, wipe pan with paper
towel, add ½ tablespoon of olive oil, and heat until almost
smoking. Add kale and sauté about thirty seconds to coat
with oil. Add about ⅓ cup of reserved noodle water to pan
and cover with a lid. Cook until kale is tender, stirring occasionally, about three minutes. Add vegetables, noodles, and

parmesan cheese, and toss all ingredients together. Add a bit more reserved noodle water if dish starts to become dry. Divide between two plates and sprinkle chives on top.

Serves 2.

*   *   *   *   *

Pesto Bluefish

PER SERVING: 750 CALORIES (KCAL) ~ 41 G FAT ~ 10 G SATURATED FAT
132 MG CHOLESTEROL ~ 58 G PROTEIN ~ 726 MG SODIUM
38 G CARBOHYDRATE ~ 10 G FIBER ~ 8 G SUGAR ~ 507 MG CALCIUM

*Basil-crusted bluefish with broccoli and tomato
sautéed with shallot and white wine*

1 12-ounce bluefish filet
2 slices white bread, crust removed and diced
1 bunch basil, cleaned and chopped
¼ cup pine nuts
2 ounces parmesan cheese, grated
1 tablespoon olive oil
Salt and pepper
½ tablespoon olive oil
1 bunch broccoli, florets removed and cut into bite-size pieces
1 tomato, seeded and chopped
Juice of 1 lemon
1 shallot, peeled and minced
1 garlic clove, thinly sliced
¼ cup dry white wine
½ tablespoon butter
Salt and freshly ground black pepper

Preheat oven to 400° F.

Place a medium-sized pot of water over a high heat with enough salt so that it tastes almost like the ocean.

In a food processor, grind the bread into fine crumbs, and set aside in a bowl. Next, process the basil and pine nuts in pulses to break the mixture down, stopping every three or four pulses to wipe down the sides with a spatula. When the mixture becomes fairly smooth, add parmesan and blend in. Next add olive oil in steady stream while machine is running. Fold mixture into bread crumbs and season with salt and pepper to taste.

Cut filet into two pieces. With the back of a spoon, smear pesto mix onto surface of the fish in an even ¼-inch layer. Place filets into a buttered pan, pesto side up, and add a few tablespoons of water. Bake in oven until cooked through and top is slightly brown, about twelve minutes.

While fish cooks, bring salted water to a boil, and add broccoli. Cook till crisp-tender (not raw and not overcooked). Heat a large sauté pan over medium-high heat. Pour about ½ tablespoon oil into sauté pan along with garlic and shallot; cook for about one minute, stirring to avoid burning. Add tomatoes and cook another minute. Add wine and allow liquid to reduce for about one minute. Remove broccoli from boiling water with a slotted spoon and place broccoli directly into sauté pan, along with tomato mixture. Add lemon juice and butter, reduce heat to medium, and swirl around until butter mounts sauce—do not overheat or butter will break. Remove pan from heat and adjust seasoning with salt and freshly ground pepper. Divide mixture between two plates and top with fish.

Serves 2.

* * * * *

Mediterranean Salmon

PER SERVING: 610 CALORIES (KCAL) ~ 36 G FAT ~ 12 G SATURATED FAT
137 MG CHOLESTEROL ~ 44 G PROTEIN ~ 229 MG SODIUM
29 G CARBOHYDRATE ~ 12 G FIBER ~ 13 G SUGAR ~ 105 MG CALCIUM

Broiled salmon with spicy ratatouille
(stewed eggplant, yellow and green squash, red peppers)

1 12-ounce salmon filet
2 tablespoons butter

½ tablespoon chopped fresh parsley
½ teaspoon fresh lemon zest
Salt and freshly ground pepper
½ tablespoon olive oil
1 small-to-medium yellow squash
1 small-to-medium zucchini
1 red bell pepper
1 medium eggplant
½ red onion
2 cloves garlic, minced
1 pinch red pepper flakes
1 pinch dried thyme
2 tablespoons tomato paste

Cut squash, zucchini, and eggplant into ½-inch cubes. Do this by cutting along the side of the vegetable ½-inch deep to produce "sheets," and cut each sheet into cubes. Discard the seedy cores. Dice onion into ½-inch pieces.

Mix butter with parsley and lemon. Add salt and pepper to taste.

Heat a medium sauté pan, covered with about ¼ tablespoon of olive oil, over medium-high heat, and add yellow squash. Season squash with salt and pepper, and lower heat to medium, making sure squash is cooked through but is not mushy. Set aside in a medium saucepan. Repeat with zucchini, eggplant, and red pepper. Over medium heat, sauté onion until translucent; add pepper flakes, thyme, and garlic. Cook one minute and add tomato paste, mixing so the paste comes into as much contact with pan's surface as possible. Fold this into the rest of the vegetables in the saucepan, and set aside over very low heat. Adjust seasoning with salt and freshly ground pepper.

Heat broiler to high. Cut fish in two, season with salt and freshly ground pepper, and place on a foil-lined sheet pan rubbed with a little olive oil. Place pan a few inches from broiler coils, and cook through on one side, allowing to brown a little on top.

Distribute ratatouille between two plates and place salmon on top. Top each piece of hot fish with compounded butter and allow to melt over fish.

Serves 2.

* * * * *

Mackerel Escabeche

PER SERVING: 700 CALORIES (KCAL) ~ 37 G FAT ~ 7 G SATURATED FAT
119 MG CHOLESTEROL ~ 48 G PROTEIN ~ 725 MG SODIUM
47 G CARBOHYDRATE ~ 12 G FIBER ~ 8 G SUGAR ~ 436 MG CALCIUM

*Spanish mackerel sautéed and then marinated
in a mixture of onions, peppers, and sherry vinegar.
Serve with spinach and wheat berry sauté*

1½ tablespoons olive oil
1 12-ounce mackerel filet
Flour for dredging
1 small red onion, thinly sliced
1 yellow or red bell pepper, sliced
¾ cup sherry vinegar
½ cup water
2 cloves garlic, sliced thin
½ tablespoon sugar
1 pinch red pepper flakes
½ cup wheat berries
1 cup water
2 teaspoons salt
2 bunches leaf spinach, trimmed and washed
Salt and freshly ground pepper

Heat wheat berries, salt, and water in a small saucepan over medium-high heat. When water starts to simmer, cover with lid and reduce heat to lowest setting. Wheat berries should cook thoroughly in about thirty-five minutes. Test and add more water if necessary.

Heat medium-sized skillet over medium-high heat. Cut fish into two even pieces, season with salt and pepper, and dredge in flour. Add about ½ tablespoon of olive oil and sauté fish on both sides until cooked through. Remove fish from pan and set aside in a pie pan or similar dish.

Add ½ tablespoon of olive oil to pan along with onions and peppers. Cook over medium heat for about three minutes or until vegetables start to soften. Drain excess oil from pan and add garlic and pepper flakes. Stir over medium-high heat for thirty seconds; deglaze with water and vinegar and add sugar. When sugar dissolves and onions are soft, pour over fish. Let sit.

Wipe sauté pan with a paper towel and return to high heat. Add about ½ tablespoon olive oil and heat to nearly smoking. Add spinach and a generous pinch of salt and sauté. When spinach is wilted, add cooked wheat berries. Spinach is finished when tender, about one minute more. Divide between two plates. Serve with marinated fish.

Serves 2.

·　·　·　·　·

Spicy Grilled Shrimp and Quinoa

PER SERVING: 664 CALORIES (KCAL) ~ 28 G FAT ~ 4 G SATURATED FAT
344 MG CHOLESTEROL ~ 56 G PROTEIN ~ 365 MG SODIUM
50 G CARBOHYDRATE ~ 13 G FIBER ~ 4 G SUGAR ~ 226 MG CALCIUM

*Shrimp dusted with spice and grilled, served with
quinoa salad with avocado, cucumber, cilantro, and lime*

¾ pound large shrimp, peeled
1 teaspoon cumin
1 teaspoon salt
½ teaspoon paprika
¼ teaspoon ground black pepper
½ cup quinoa
1½ cups water
½ teaspoon salt
1 cucumber
3 scallions

1 avocado
1 lime
¼ cup chopped cilantro
1 tablespoon olive oil
Salt and pepper
Romaine lettuce, chopped (a couple of handfuls)
Lime wedges

Mix cumin, salt, paprika, and black pepper.

Rinse quinoa with cold water. Place into a small saucepan, along with 1½ cups water and salt. Bring to a boil, cover, and reduce heat to low. Quinoa will be ready in twelve to fifteen minutes. Remove lid and fluff with a fork.

Peel cucumber, slice in half lengthwise, and remove seeds with a spoon. Dice halves into ¼-inch pieces.

Clean scallions and slice green and white parts thinly crosswise; discard roots at the base.

Cut avocado in half around pit. Pull apart, remove pit, and separate skin from halves with a large spoon. Dice avocado halves into ¼-inch pieces, and immediately toss with lime juice. Add to cooked quinoa, along with cucumber, scallions, and cilantro. Fluff in olive oil and add salt and freshly ground pepper to taste.

Heat a large skillet over medium-high heat; add about ½ tablespoon olive oil and swirl it around in the pan. Toss shrimp with spice mixture and add shrimp to pan, one at a time, gently pressing shrimp onto pan surface. Allow to sear about 1½ minutes or until shrimp turns pink. Flip and finish cooking. Line two plates with romaine lettuce; place half of quinoa mixture in center of each plate, and arrange shrimp around the salad. Serve with additional lime wedges.

Serves 2.

·   ·   ·   ·   ·

Steak with Creamed Spinach and Millet Croquettes

PER SERVING: 635 CALORIES (KCAL) ~ 24 G FAT ~ 8 G SATURATED FAT
163 MG CHOLESTEROL ~ 72 G PROTEIN ~ 619 MG SODIUM
34 G CARBOHYDRATE ~ 10 G FIBER ~ 2 G SUGAR ~ 563 MG CALCIUM

*Your favorite steak simply prepared and combined
with a healthy dose of spinach and millet*

4 6-ounce beef steaks (cut of your choice),
prepared according to your desired method
4 bunches curly spinach, washed and trimmed
¼ cup cream
Salt and pepper
½ cup millet
2 cups water
3 scallions, washed and chopped
1 clove garlic, minced
1 red bell pepper, diced into small pieces
1 teaspoon Worcestershire sauce
1 dash Tabasco sauce
1 egg, lightly beaten
2 ounces parmesan, grated
¼ cup all-purpose flour
1½ tablespoons olive oil

Fill large pot with water and bring to a boil. Add enough salt
so that the water tastes almost like the ocean. Add spinach
and cook until tender, about two minutes after water returns
to a boil. Remove spinach and plunge into cold water.
Squeeze spinach dry and put into processor. Pulse until
spinach breaks up evenly, scraping down sides. When fairly
uniform, run processor continuously and add cream in a
steady stream. Add salt and freshly ground pepper to taste.

Bring millet and water to a boil, cover, and simmer until
liquid is gone, about one-half hour. Set aside and let rest.

Pour about ½ tablespoon olive oil into a sauté pan, and
sauté peppers, combined with scallions, until soft. Add garlic

and cook thirty seconds more. Fluff millet with a fork; add scallion mixture, Tabasco, Worcestershire sauce, egg, parmesan, and flour, and combine. Add salt and pepper to taste. Form mixture into balls the size of golf balls and flatten into disks. Heat skillet with remaining olive oil and cook until brown. Flip and put in oven for twelve minutes or until cooked through. Serve on platter with reheated creamed spinach and steaks.

Serves 4.

. . . . .

Southern Stuffed Pork Chops and Red Flannel Hash

PER SERVING: 542 CALORIES (KCAL) ~ 23 G FAT ~ 9 G SATURATED FAT
123 MG CHOLESTEROL ~ 44 G PROTEIN ~ 640 MG SODIUM
30 G CARBOHYDRATE ~ 5 G FIBER ~ 10 G SUGAR ~ 119 MG CALCIUM

Pork chops stuffed with Swiss chard and served with hash made from sweet potatoes, beets, and bacon

4 6-ounce pork chops
1 bunch Swiss chard
1 tablespoon olive oil
2 red onions, chopped, divided into two parts
1 clove garlic, minced
2 tablespoons white vinegar
1 dash Tabasco
¼ cup cream
2 tablespoons bulgur
¾ cup white wine
½ tablespoon cornstarch
1 tablespoon water
2 medium sweet potatoes
2 medium beets
4 slices bacon
¼ cup sour cream
2 tablespoons Dijon mustard
⅛ cup chopped parsley
Salt and pepper

Preheat oven to 375° F.

Wash and dry beets and sweet potatoes. Prick all around with a knife, rub with olive oil, season with salt and pepper, and wrap in foil. Place into oven and cook until knife is easily inserted, about an hour.

Set a medium-sized pan filled with water over high heat and bring water to a boil. Trim and wash Swiss chard in a large bowl of cold water, shake dry, and chop into two-inch pieces. Add enough salt to boiling water so that it tastes almost like the ocean, and add Swiss chard. Cook until tender, about four to six minutes. Drain chard from pot and plunge into ice-cold water.

Place a sauté pan over medium heat; add ½ tablespoon olive oil and half the onions. Cook until onions are translucent. Add garlic and turn up heat to medium high. Cook garlic for about thirty seconds, stirring constantly, and then add chard. Cook another minute and add vinegar. After vinegar reduces (about a minute), add cream and bulgur. Stir until thickened, about three minutes, and set aside to cool.

With a small knife, cut into center of each pork chop on the end opposite the bone. Once knife is inserted, pivot it carefully from side to side, avoiding breaking all the way through, to make a pocket. Stuff each pocket with ¼ of the stuffing, and close pocket with toothpicks.

Heat ½ tablespoon olive oil in an ovenproof sauté pan just large enough to hold the chops. Season chops with salt and pepper and sear on each side until browned. Remove chops from pan and deglaze with wine. Once wine is reduced by half, turn off heat, return chops to pan, and cover pan with foil. Place in oven and cook to desired doneness, being careful not to dry out chops. (Start checking after twenty minutes.)

Peel cooled sweet potatoes and beets. Dice into ¼-inch pieces, and mix with parsley, mustard, and sour cream. Add salt and pepper to taste. Cook bacon in skillet until crisp, and crumble into mixture. Pour mixture into pan with bacon drippings, spread evenly, and cook over medium-high heat until crisp. Flip and crisp on other side.

Remove chops from oven and return to stove over medium-high heat. Combine cornstarch with water to make a slurry, and whisk into juices to make a gravy. Gravy will thicken when it reaches a boil. Cook another minute and adjust seasoning.

Divide hash among four plates, place a chop on each, and serve with gravy.

Serves 4.

. . . .
                    .
                    .

FACE Program Exercises

To put it very simply, the FACE program exercises nourish and stimulate your body's natural process of connective-tissue repair and rejuvenation. They can improve circulation to the skin and other connective tissues, thus delivering more nutrients and removing more waste products and helping to prevent new connective-tissue problems from surfacing in the future.

HOW DO THE FACE PROGRAM EXERCISES WORK?

The diet, exercise, and flexibility portions of the program form the foundation that promotes a healthy balance of connective-tissue turnover. Dietary supplements provide the most concentrated source of the metabolic regulators and connective-tissue building blocks that the body needs to support optimal turnover, synthesis, and repair. The combined effects of exercise, stretching, proper nutrition, and supplementation result in an ideal environment to promote connective-tissue health.

These exercises are a simple and effective approach to maintaining your body's vast array of connective tissues, including those in your skin. By maintaining proper function and supporting the body's vital renewal processes, the exercises can help you confront the daily wear and tear your skin encounters. The main goal is for you to learn how you can take meaningful steps every day that will help you achieve and maintain a healthy, active lifestyle—and in doing so promote the health not just of your skin but of all your connective tissues.

PERFORM FACE MOVEMENTS
ON A DAILY BASIS

It's up to you to decide whether to perform these movements before or after your other exercise regimen. Sometimes you might find that they serve as a nice warm-up for your walking or other exercise regimens (such as strength training), and on other days they can serve as a relaxing cool-down (say, if you take up jogging or aerobics). No matter when you do them, the important thing is that you *do them on a regular basis* to provide the constant stimulation, stretching, strengthening, balancing, hydration, oxygenation, and rejuvenation your skin needs.

Perform each movement only within a comfortable range; you should not feel any pain or discomfort. If any movement is uncomfortable to the point of pain, do not do it. Of course, you will want to challenge yourself a bit and provide a stretching stimulus to your connective tissues, but it is important to stay within your own personal comfort range with each movement. There are no prizes for pushing yourself too far—and doing so may actually increase your risk of injury and tissue damage.

Hold each movement for thirty to sixty seconds; the whole series of ten movements will take between five and ten minutes. This is certainly not a great investment of time, especially given the wide range of circulatory, flexibility, and stress-management benefits that you'll enjoy in a very short period of time.

The only equipment you need is a yoga mat or a beach towel and clothes that allow you to move freely. Are you ready? Let's go!

1. Child's Pose

This is one of the classic yoga poses—a resting and starting pose that serves as the base from which many other poses and stretches emanate. We'll use it as the initial movement because it helps awaken and stimulate each of the major body parts that we'll target with the subsequent movements.

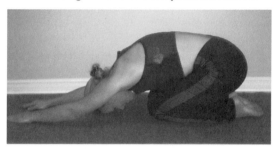

From a standing position, move to your hands and knees. Point your toes so that the tops of your feet are flat on the floor and your derrière rests on your heels. Place your hands flat on the mat, about shoulder-width apart. Slowly reach forward, extending your arms straight out in front of you. Lengthen your back and try to place your forehead as close to the floor as is comfortable. When you reach your farthest comfortable point, breathe slowly and deeply. Hold this position for thirty to sixty seconds.

2. Arch

This movement is sometimes called "the Cat," and it resembles a modified version of a standard yoga pose known as Downward Facing Dog. You can move directly into the Arch position from the Child's Pose—or you can pause, take a breath, and start again from your hands and knees, as described below.

From a position on your hands and knees, place your hands shoulder-width apart and directly beneath your shoulders. To a count of five, slowly arch your back upward (as a scared cat might arch its back) and point your head downward, gently tucking your chin. Hold for a count of five as you reach your highest arch point. Slowly arch your back downward and move your head upward using the same five-second count, and again pause at your lowest arch point for a count of five. Continue breathing deeply through three full repetitions of arching up and down, for a total duration of sixty seconds.

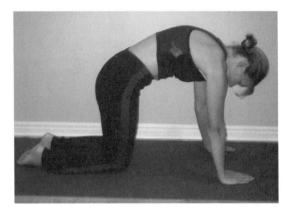

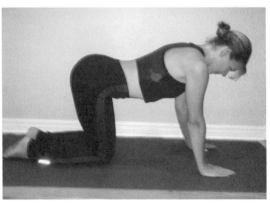

3. Cobra

This position is sometime called the Lizard and is similar to the Upward Facing Dog pose in traditional yoga practice. Aside from the obvious advantage to overall flexibility, the Cobra movement serves to open up and expand your entire front torso, an effect that will greatly improve your ability to breathe and thus to deliver vital oxygen to the repair processes in every tissue.

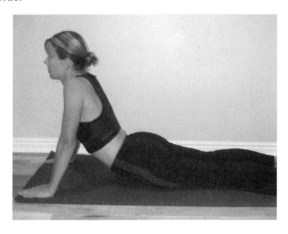

Lying face down on your mat, place the palms of your hands under your shoulders. Inhale slowly and deeply, hold for a moment and then, while slowly exhaling, push up from your hands, raising your head and shoulders and allowing your lower back to arch naturally. Arch up as high as comfort allows, continue breathing slowly and deeply, and hold for thirty to sixty seconds. Slowly return to the beginning, face-down position. As you become more comfortable with the Cobra movement, you will find it easier to push yourself into a fuller arch. For a more advanced position, you can try arching your neck backward to look toward the ceiling.

4. Squat

Okay—time to teach your skeleton what proper alignment feels like. This squat position is actually the resting position that is most natural in terms of skeletal alignment. Sitting in a chair (as most of us do for hours every day) is one of the worst biomechanical positions—not only because of the extreme

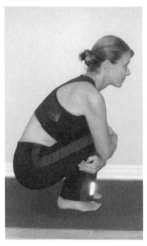

pressures that sitting delivers to the back but also because it interferes with optimal breathing. You'll be amazed by how much deeper and fuller each breath is when you learn to maintain proper skeletal alignment. The Squat helps to realign your entire body into a more natural position.

Start in a standing position with your feet about shoulder-width apart and your toes pointing straight ahead. Take a deep breath and slowly squat down, bringing your derrière toward the backs of your ankles. Your hands can hang by your sides, or you can wrap them around your knees or place them on the ground in front or to the side to help balance yourself. Continue to breathe slowly and deeply, and hold this position for thirty to sixty seconds. As your balance improves in the Squat, you will find that you can maintain this comfortable position for many minutes without using your hands for balance or support.

5. Sky Reach

Also known as the Pillar Stretch or the Mountain Pose in yoga, this movement can be done seated or standing. I prefer to do the Sky Reach seated with legs crossed (as pictured) because I feel that it provides a better stretch in the seated position and a very noticeable opening of the airways, leading to better breathing and oxygenation of the blood. The choice is yours; you may wish to experiment with both seated and standing positions to see which you prefer.

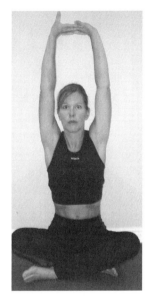

From a cross-legged seated position (or standing with feet shoulder-width apart, toes pointing straight ahead), inhale slowly and deeply. Interlace your fingers, turn your palms away from your body, and reach your hands toward the sky. Keep your shoulders pointed downward, rather than allowing them to creep up toward your ears. Look straight ahead, keep your spine straight, and breathe slowly and deeply. Hold your most comfortably extended position for thirty to sixty seconds.

6. Figure 8

Also called the Pretzel and the Seated Hip Twist in some forms of yoga, the Figure 8 is one of my personal favorites. As a runner and cyclist, my hips and lower back are in a constant state of stress, so this movement is vital to maintaining optimal flexibility and mobility in these important "core" areas. Tightness in these core areas of your body can quickly lead to subtle changes in how you breathe—and ultimately in how much oxygen you're able to deliver to your skin and other connective tissues. In addition, you'll simply feel better and more relaxed throughout your entire body if your core muscles are limber and flexible.

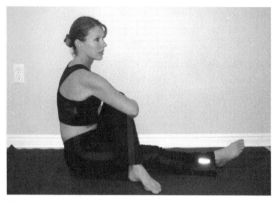

From a seated position with your legs extended straight in front of you, keep your right leg straight and cross your left foot over to the outside of your right knee. Grasp the outside of your left knee and gently twist your torso, while pulling the left knee toward the ribs on your right side. Keep your back straight, rather than allowing it to hunch over. You can do this by imagining a string attached to the crown of your head, gently pulling upward. Continue breathing slowly and deeply until you feel a stretch in your left hip, derrière, and lower back. Hold for twenty to thirty seconds. Slowly release the stretch, extend your left leg, bend the right leg, and repeat the movement on the opposite side.

7. Cross Twist

This position is in two parts—starting with a very simple knee-to-chest movement that you may have performed as a child in gym class, followed by the twisting position that is sometimes called a T-Roll or a Crucifix Twist because of the position of your upper body and arms during the movement.

Lying on your back with both legs extended straight outward, use both hands to bring your right knee up to your chest. Take a deep breath, and with your hands gently clasping your knee and shin, slowly pull your right leg/knee into your chest

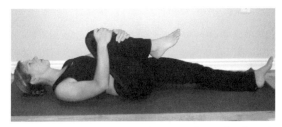

until you can feel a gentle stretch in your lower back and right hip. Pull as far as feels comfortable, and hold this position for fifteen to thirty seconds while you continue to breathe slowly and deeply.

At the end of your hold, slowly extend your hands out toward your sides, forming a "T" shape with your body. Slowly rotate your pelvis and torso as you lower your right knee toward your left side, bringing the inside of your right knee as close to the mat as possible while keeping both palms and shoulders flat on the mat. In your most comfortable twist position, continue to breathe slowly and deeply, and hold for fifteen to thirty seconds. Repeat both positions (knee-to-chest and twist) with your left leg.

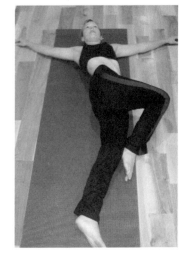

As you become more flexible and can pull your leg/knee closer to your chest and lower your knee closer to the mat, you may also begin to feel a gentle stretch in your opposite hip flexor (the front part of your hip, an area that becomes very tight in many people and causes tension throughout the body, accompanied by restricted breathing).

8. Superman

Also known in some forms of yoga as the Locust position and in Pilates as the Swimmer, the Superman position is popular as much for its strengthening and balancing qualities as for its flexibility and breathing benefits. It can be performed in several variations, from easy to advanced, depending on your degree of flexibility.

Start from a position lying face down, forehead flat on the mat. Arms should be stretched out in front of you with your palms flat on the floor. Breathe slowly and deeply for a few moments. Keeping your forehead flat on the mat, slowly raise *both* your *right* hand/arm and *left* foot/leg off of the mat as far as comfort allows. You should feel a slight stretch in your front torso and through your entire back, hip, and derrière region. If you feel any lower-back pain at all, you should lower your hand and/or foot until you feel comfortable again. Continue taking slow, deep breaths and hold this extended position for fifteen to thirty seconds. Slowly lower your right hand and left foot, take a deep breath in the beginning (face-down) position, and repeat the movement with your left hand and right foot.

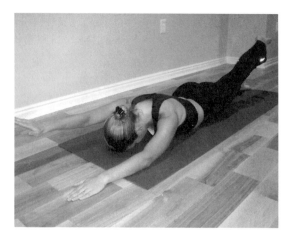

9. Plank

This movement is a classic yoga position that helps integrate upper- and lower-body alignment. You can think of the Plank as a static push-up in both high and low positions. We start this movement with the high position and progress to the low position. In doing so, we encourage muscle activity in all parts of the body, which stimulates circulation and delivery of nutrients to the skin and a range of connective tissues. Breathing is an especially important consideration in this movement, because with so many muscles being activated, you'll have to concentrate on full, deep breaths during the entire movement.

Start from the same relaxed face-down position as the Superman movement (see exercise #8). Place your hands palm down, directly under your shoulders. Take a deep, cleansing breath and fully extend your arms, pushing up to the high Plank position. Try to stay up on your toes while you maintain a straight spine and neck and focus your eyes on the floor directly in front of your fingertips. Concentrate on maintaining slow, deep, even breaths as you hold this position for fifteen to thirty seconds. Don't allow your hips to pike upward. Visualize a long, straight line running from the back of your head to your heels. This can be a very challenging movement, especially if you lack upper-body strength, so only maintain this high position for as long as you feel comfortable. Then move

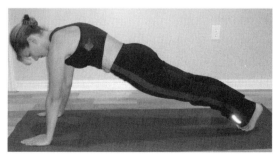

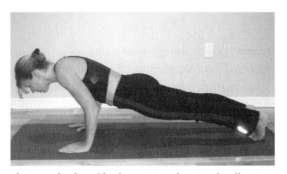

directly into the low Plank position, by simply allowing your arms to slowly bend and bringing your elbows to the sides of your torso while keeping your body and legs a few inches off the floor. Engage your abdominal muscles to prevent your spine from arching downward into a sway-backed position. Keep aiming for that long, straight line running down your back. Continuing to breathe slowly and deeply, hold this position for fifteen to thirty seconds (or however long you can maintain good form) before slowly returning to your starting position resting on the mat. Take another deep, cleansing breath.

10. Multi-Split

This position is another two-part movement that simultaneously targets circulation in multiple body parts, while at the same time improving muscle strength and balance. The primary idea behind this movement is to get the connective tissues in the upper and lower body aligned and working in concert with one another. In some forms of yoga, this movement is known as the Stork or the Tree, and sometimes as the Crescent Lunge, depending on the direction of the movement.

Start in a standing position, with your toes pointing straight ahead and your arms at your sides. Take a deep, cleansing breath. In the first part of the movement, extend your arms upward and away from your sides, so they are parallel to the floor. Then bring the sole of your right foot slowly up the inside of your left leg, raising your right foot as high as feels comfortable. Keep your hips level. Continue maintaining a slow, deep, rhythmic breathing pattern (and your balance!) as you hold this position for fifteen to thirty seconds. Slowly return your right foot to the floor and repeat on the other side.

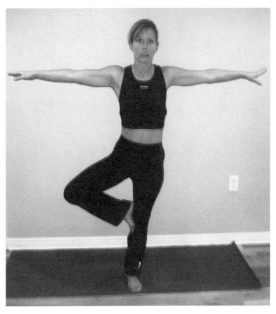

In the second part of the movement, you will start from the same position (standing, with toes forward and arms at sides). Take a deep, cleansing breath, look straight ahead, and step forward with your right foot. Keeping both knees pointing straight ahead, bend your right knee into as deep a lunge as you feel comfortable with. Use a wide stance so that your bent knee doesn't go past your toes, which could result in hyper-flexion of your knee. If necessary, adjust your position by stepping out a little farther with your right foot. Continue your

slow, deep-breathing process, while you reach your arms upward, straight over your head. Keep your shoulders down.
Imagine lengthening your spine from your low back all the
way up to the ceiling with each breath. Hold this position for
fifteen to thirty seconds before slowly returning your arms to

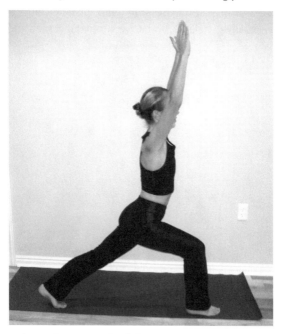

your sides and stepping back from your lunge into your starting position. Repeat with your left leg.

After finishing this last movement, you should come back
to a resting position for a few last deep, cleansing breaths. You
can use a comfortable standing position, the Squat position,
or even the Child's Pose to bring everything to a relaxing conclusion. Experiment with each option to find out how you
prefer to end your sessions—or try ending with a different position each time.

ENGAGE IN REGULAR EXERCISE

Exercise is a vital part of achieving and maintaining healthy connective tissue. Whether we're talking about skin or any other collagen-containing connective tissue (muscles, tendons, ligaments, etc.), the right amount of the right type of exercise can help stimulate production of new collagen, removal of damaged tissue, and delivery of vital oxygen and nutrients. Just as proper exercise can promote connective-tissue health, inadequate or excessive levels of exercise can lead to unhealthy connective tissue by accelerating damage and delaying repair.

Our bodies are designed to move. One famous philosopher commented that the human body is the only machine that breaks down from *underuse* rather than from overuse (but your body can break down from overuse as well, as evidenced by the numerous overtrained athletes I have worked with throughout the years). In many ways the *motion* of exercise, or any type of physical activity, can be thought of as *lotion* for your connective tissues. The simple act of moving your body helps to hydrate skin and stimulate tissue repair, while sitting around like a couch potato sends a constant "breakdown" signal (called "atrophy") that leads to thinning, wrinkling, and drying of skin tissues.

But, you might ask, what is the "best" exercise to do? The answer is "Anything you like"—whether it be the simple act of walking or something more complex such as aerobics classes or weight lifting or skydiving (just kidding). Take walking, for example. A number of studies show that walking at a moderate pace for twenty minutes daily can reduce your risk of a variety of diseases—largely due to the enhanced circulation, nutrient delivery, and waste-product removal it provides.

Walking is a pretty simple exercise; it doesn't require any fancy or expensive equipment and you can do it virtually anywhere. That said, you'll want to make sure that you have a pair of comfortable and supportive shoes, as well as a "thumbs-up" from your health-care provider indicating that it's okay for you to engage in a moderate-to-vigorous exercise regimen.

In good weather, you can walk outside and enjoy the sights and sounds of your neighborhood or a local park. In bad weather, you can walk around the mall (many shopping malls have organized walking groups that meet before the stores open and the mall gets crowded with shoppers). When you get comfortable with walking on a regular basis, you can vary the route and the intensity (walking faster or slower and adding hills or flats). Walking can also become a part of your mental exercise as much as it is your physical exercise because it can allow you some time to get away and de-stress while your mind (and your body) wanders.

The flexibility movements, the Helping Hand diet, and the physical activity that you'll be doing as part of the FACE program will all help to control stress and reduce cortisol exposure. Even letting your mind go for the five to ten minutes while you're performing the flexibility movements will be beneficial for stress control. The Helping Hand diet will help to take the guesswork and associated stress out of meal planning and calorie counting. The physical activity, whether it's walking or another form of exercise, should be viewed as *your* time that you invest in mental and physical health—and you should do *something* on as many days of the week as you possibly can. You should also keep in mind that stress is a very individual phenomenon; what stresses you out may be no big deal to someone else (and vice versa). This makes your approach to stress management a personal and individualized process that requires you to identify your own specific stressors and your own specific solutions for dealing with them.

References

Alberts, D., J. Ranger-Moore, J. Einspahr, K. Saboda, P. Bozzo, Y. Liu, XC Xu, R. Lotan, J. Warneke, S. Salasche, S. Stratton, N. Levine, R. Goldman, M. Islas, L. Duckett, D. Thompson, P. Bartels, and J. Foote. 2004. Safety and efficacy of dose-intensive oral vitamin A in subjects with sun-damaged skin. *Clinical Cancer Research* 10(6): 1875–1880.

Alesci, S., and S.R. Bornstein. 2000. Neuroimmunoregulation of androgens in the adrenal gland and the skin. *Hormone Research* 54(5–6): 281–286.

Belch, J.J., and A. Hill. 2000. Evening primrose oil and borage oil in rheumatologic conditions. *American Journal of Clinical Nutrition* 71(1 Suppl): 352S–356S.

Berking, C. 2005. [The role of ultraviolet irradiation in malignant melanoma.] (Article in German) *Hautarzt* 56(7): 687–696.

Bernkop-Schnurch, A., et al. 2004. Development of a sustained release dosage form for alpha-lipoic acid. II. Evaluation in human volunteers. *Drug Development and Industrial Pharmacy.* 30(1): 35–42.

Blaha, J., and I. Pondelicek. 1997. Prevention and therapy of postburn scars. *ACTA Chirurgiae Plasticae* 39(1): 17–21.

Boelsma, E., et al. 2001. Nutritional skin care: Health effects of micronutrients and fatty acids. *American Journal of Clinical Nutrition* 73(5): 853–864.

Bosset, S., et al. 2003. Photoaging shows histological features of chronic skin inflammation without clinical and molecular abnormalities. *British Journal of Dermatology* 149(4): 826–835.

Boule, N.G., et al. 2005. Effects of exercise training on glucose homeostasis: The HERITAGE Family Study. *Diabetes Care* 28(1): 108–114.

Buss, I.C., et al. 1997. The effectiveness of massage in preventing pressure sores: A literature review. *Rehabilitation Nursing* 22(5): 229–234, 242.

Cappel, M., D. Mauger, and D. Thiboutot. Correlation between serum levels of insulin-like growth factor 1, dehydroepiandrosterone sulfate, and dihydrotestosterone and acne lesion counts in adult women. *Archives of Dermatology* 141(3): 333–338.

Castaneda, C. 2003. Diabetes control with physical activity and exercise. *Nutrition in Clinical Care* 6(2): 89–96.

Catani, M.V., et al. 2005. Biological role of vitamin C in keratinocytes. *Nutrition Reviews* 63(3): 81–90.

Chen, K., et al. 2005. Oral retinoids for the prevention of skin cancers in solid organ transplant recipients: A systematic review of randomized controlled trials. *British Journal of Dermatology* 152(3): 518–523.

Chen, Y.Y., and P.S. Rabinovitch. 1990. Altered cell cycle responses to insulin-like growth factor 1, but not platelet-derived growth factor and epidermal growth factor, in senescing human fibroblasts. *Journal of Cellular Physiology* 144(1): 18–25.

Chivot, M. 2005. Retinoid therapy for acne: A comparative review. *American Journal of Clinical Dermatology* 6(1): 13–19.

Clarke, N., et al. 2004. Retinoids: Potential in cancer prevention and therapy. *Expert Reviews in Molecular Medicine* 6(25): 1–23.

DeGroot, J. 2004. The AGE of the matrix: Chemistry, consequence and cure. *Current Opinions in Pharmacology* 4(3): 301–305.

Ebrecht, M., et al. 2004. Perceived stress and cortisol levels predict speed of wound healing in healthy male adults. *Psychoneuroendocrinology* 29(6): 798–809.

Eleftheriou, C.S., et al. 1991. Cellular aging related proteins secreted by human fibroblasts. *Mutation Research/DNA Repair* 256(2–6): 127–138.

Frank, L.L., et al. 2005. Effects of exercise on metabolic risk variables in overweight postmenopausal women: A randomized clinical trial. *Obesity Research* 13(3): 615–625.

Fuchs, J., et al. 2003. HPLC analysis of vitamin E isoforms in human epidermis: Correlation with minimal erythema dose and free radical scavenging activity. *Free Radical Biology and Medicine* 34(3): 330–336.

Fung, T.T., et al. 2002. Intake of alcohol and alcoholic beverages and the risk of basal cell carcinoma of the skin. *Cancer Epidemiology, Biomarkers & Prevention* 11(10 Pt 1): 1119–1122.

Giacomoni, P.U., and G. Rein. 2001. Factors of skin aging share common mechanisms. *Biogerontology* 2(4): 219–229.

Grossman, R. 2005. The role of dimethylaminoethanol in cosmetic dermatology. *American Journal of Clinical Dermatology* 6(1): 39–47.

Hinds, T., et al. 2004. Effects of massage on limb and skin blood flow after quadriceps exercise. *Medicine and Science in Sports and Exercise* 36(8): 1308–1313.

Horrobin, D.F. 2000. Essential fatty acid metabolism and its modification in atopic eczema. *American Journal of Clinical Nutrition* 71(1Suppl): 367S–372S.

Horswell, B.B. 1998. Scar modification: Techniques for revision and camouflage. *Atlas of the Oral and Maxillofacial Surgery Clinics of North America* 6(2): 55–72.

Hsu, S. 2005. Green tea and the skin. *Journal of the American Academy of Dermatology* 52(6): 1049–1059.

Humbert, P.G., et al. 2003. Topical ascorbic acid on photoaged skin. Clinical, topographical and ultrastructural evaluation: Double-blind study vs. placebo. *Experimental Dermatology* 12(3): 237–244.

Iida, I., and K. Noro. 1995. An analysis of the reduction of elasticity on the aging of human skin and the recovering effect of a facial massage. *Ergonomics*. 38(9): 1921–1931.

Jain, S.K., and G. Lim. 2000. Lipoic acid decreases lipid peroxidation and protein glycosylation and increases (Na(+) + K (+))- and Ca(++)-ATPase activities in high glucose-treated human erythrocytes. *Free Radical Biology and Medicine* 29(11): 1122–1128.

Jeanmaire, C., et al. 2001. Glycation during human dermal intrinsic and actinic aging: An in vivo and in vitro model study. *British Journal of Dermatology* 145(1): 10–18.

Kagan, V.E., et al. 1992. Dihydrolipoic acid—a universal antioxidant both in the membrane and in the aqueous phase. Reduction of peroxyl, ascorbyl and chromanoxyl radicals. *Biochemical Pharmacology* 44(8): 1637–1649.

Katiyar, S.K. 2003. Skin photoprotection by green tea: Antioxidant and immunomodulatory effects. *Current Drug Targets: Immune, Endocrine and Metabolic Disorders* 3(3): 234–242.

Konrad, T., et al. 1999. Alpha-lipoic acid treatment decreases serum lactate and pyruvate concentrations and improves glucose effectiveness in lean and obese patients with type 2 diabetes. *Diabetes Care* 22(2): 280–287.

Krug, M., et al. 2004. [Addiction to tobacco and the consequences for the skin.] (Article in German) *Hautarzt* 55(3): 301–315; quiz 316.

Meaume, S., and P. Senet. 1999. Prevention of decubitus scars in the elderly. *Presse Medicale* 28(33): 1846–1853.

Miller, P.L. 2005. *The life extension revolution: The new science of growing older without aging.* New York: Bantam Dell.

Nachbar, F., and H.C. Korting. 1995. The role of vitamin E in normal and damaged skin. *Journal of Molecular Medicine* 73(1): 7–17.

Nola, I., and L. Kotrulja. 2003. Skin photodamage and lifetime photoprotection. *Acta Dermatovenerologica Croatica* 11(1): 32–40.

Packer, L., et al. 2001. Molecular aspects of alpha-tocotrienol antioxidant action and cell signaling. *Journal of Nutrition* 131(2): 369S–373S.

Perricone, N.V. 2004. *The Perricone promise: Look younger, live longer in three easy steps.* New York: Warner Books.

Puglia, C., S. Tropea, L Rizza, N.A. Santagati, and F. Bonina. 2005. In vitro percutaneous adsorption studies and in vivo evaluation of anti-inflammatory activity of essential fatty acids (EFA) from fish oil extracts. *International Journal of Pharmaceutics* 299(1–2): 41–48.

Raychaudhuri, S.P., and J. Gross. 2000. Psoriasis risk factors: Role of lifestyle practices. *Cutis* 66(5): 348–352.

Rutter, K., et al. 2003. Green tea extract suppresses the age-related increase in collagen cross-linking and fluorescent products in C57BL/6 mice. *International Journal for Vitamin and Nutrition Research* 73(6): 453–460.

Saladi, R.N., and A.N. Persaud. 2005. The causes of skin cancer: A comprehensive review. *Drugs Today* 41(1): 37–53.

Schaffer, S., et al. 2005. Tocotrienols: Constitutional effects in aging and disease. *Journal of Nutrition* 135(2): 151–154.

Shankar, J., et al. 2002. Management of peri-ocular skin tumours by laissez-faire technique: Analysis of functional and cosmetic results. *Eye* 16(1): 50–53.

Simopoulos, A.P. 2002. The importance of the ratio of omega-6/omega-3 essential fatty acids. *Biomedicine and Pharmacotherapy* 56(8): 365–379.

Spiclin, P., et al. 2003. Sodium ascorbyl phosphate in topical microemulsions. *International Journal of Pharmaceutics* 256(1–2): 65–73.

Stratigos, A.J., and A.D. Katsambas. 2005. The role of topical retinoids in the treatment of photoaging. *Drugs* 65(8): 1061–1072.

Talbott, S. 2003. *A guide to understanding dietary supplements.* Binghamton, NY: The Haworth Press.

Taylor, S.C. 2002. Skin of color: Biology, structure, function, and implications for dermatologic disease. *Journal of the American Academy of Dermatology* 46(2Suppl): S41–S62.

Thirunavukkarasu, V., et al. 2004. Lipoic acid attenuates hypertension and improves insulin sensitivity, kallikrein activity and nitrite levels in high fructose-fed rats. *Journal of Comparative Physiology [B]* 174(8): 587–592.

———. 2004. Fructose diet-induced skin collagen abnormalities are prevented by lipoic acid. *Experimental Diabesity Research* 5(4): 237–244.

———. 2005. Lipoic acid prevents collagen abnormalities in tail tendon of high-fructose-fed rats. *Diabetes and Obesity Metabolism* 7(3): 294–297.

Traikovich, S.S. 1999. Use of topical ascorbic acid and its effects on photodamaged skin topography. *Archives of Otolaryngology—Head and Neck Surgery* 125(10): 1091–1098.

Turaclar, U.T., et al. 1998. Effect of acute exercise on skin potential in sedentaries and trained athletes. *Indian Journal of Physiology and Pharmacology* 42(3): 369–374.

Uhoda, I., et al. 2002. Split-face study on the cutaneous tensile effect of 2-dimethylaminoethanol (deanol) gel. *Skin Research Technology* 8(3): 164–167.

Vasan, S., et al. 2003. Therapeutic potential of breakers of advanced glycation end product-protein cross-links. *Archives of Biochemistry and Biophysics* 419(1): 89–96.

Wang, S.Y., and H. Jiao. 2000. Scavenging capacity of berry crops on superoxide radicals, hydrogen peroxide, hydroxyl radicals, and singlet oxygen. *Journal of Agricultural and Food Chemistry* 48(11): 5677–5684.

Resources

Author's Books and Websites

The Cortisol Connection: Why Stress Makes You Fat and Ruins Your Health — and What You Can Do about It (Alameda, CA: Hunter House, 2002).

The Cortisol Connection Diet: The Breakthrough Program to Control Stress and Lose Weight (Alameda, CA: Hunter House, 2004).

Cortisol Connection website: www.cortisolconnection.com

Supplement Watch website: www.supplementwatch.com

To Contact the Experts Quoted in Chapter 11

Marianne Damhuis: (415) 260-3721

Shelley Rosenfeld: Conscious Skin and Body Care, (510) 551-8834, www.consciousskinandbody.com

Elina Fedatova: (312) 274-3474, elina@elinaskincare.com, www.ElinaSkinCare.com

John Nieters: (510) 814-6900, www.johnnieters.com

Karen Burke: (212) 754-1100

Other Related Websites

Eminence Organics (natural skin-care products): www.eminenceorganics.com

Websites for looking up ingredients in cosmetics: www.safecosmetics.org *and* www.ewg.org

Index